The
Twelfth
Raven

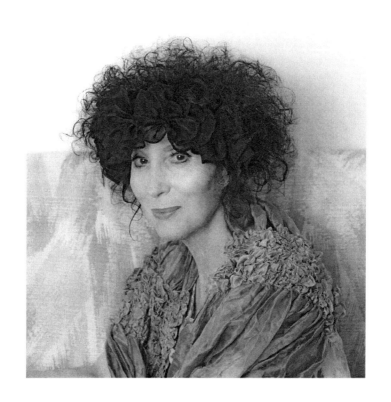

The Twelfth Raven

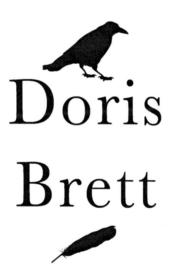

Doris Brett

A memoir of stroke,
love and recovery

UWA PUBLISHING

First published in 2014 by
UWA Publishing
Crawley, Western Australia 6009
www.uwap.uwa.edu.au

UWAP is an imprint of UWA Publishing
a division of The University of Western Australia

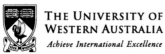

THE UNIVERSITY OF
WESTERN AUSTRALIA
Achieve International Excellence

A full CIP data entry is available from the National Library of Australia.

Cover design by Anna Maley-Fadgyas
Typeset in Bembo by Lasertype
Printed by Griffin Press

For Martin and Amantha
the loving core of my life

One for bad news,
Two for mirth,
Three is a wedding,
Four is a birth,
Five is for riches,
Six is a thief,
Seven, a journey,
Eight is for grief,
Nine is a secret,
Ten is for sorrow,
Eleven is for love,
Twelve – joy for tomorrow.

(Old English rhyme used to interpret raven sightings.)

Part 1

6 June 2009

It is a cold, cloudy morning in June when my husband Martin and I leave the house carrying three bags between us. We are heading for Frankston, nearly an hour away, for a daylong dance workshop. In the bags, we have three pairs of shoes – one for slippery floors, one for sticky, one for medium. Clothes to accommodate the weather – warm overlays for the winter outside, peel-off layers for the changed internal temperatures of dancing. Water bottles to drink from, bananas to snack on, an audio book to listen to as we drive up. We are prepared for everything. Absolutely everything. Except for what happens.

It is cold in the hall but the choreographer is taking us through our paces and we begin to warm up. It takes concentration to master the constant stream of new sequences and steps but it is also exhilarating. We are negotiating a complicated new partner dance when Martin says to me, 'It's so cold, I'm stuttering'. I nod absently although I don't hear him stuttering. Perhaps it is that cold for him? Even though it isn't.

When Alice, sitting bored at a picnic, first sees the White Rabbit, he is talking to himself. Alice is unimpressed. For some reason, she is not struck by the knowledge that rabbits cannot talk. It is only when the White Rabbit takes out a pocket watch and mutters 'I'm late! I'm late!' that she sits up and pays attention – rabbits don't have pocket watches, she thinks, something is going on. It is 10.30 am on Saturday 6 June 2009. Like Alice, I am not paying attention. And it is late. It is late.

The pocket-watch episode occurs for me just after 2.00 pm. We have been having lunch with a group of other dancers. Martin has been relatively silent but then he often is, nothing unusual in that. He is frustrated by the long lunch hour. Martin wants to be dancing. He gets up to communicate this to the organisers at another table.

He comes back soon after, looking puzzled. 'I'm having trouble putting words together', he says. And I sit up. I am a psychologist. I've studied neuropsychology. I know that not being able to put words together means something is going on. In the brain. And I don't want to know that. These things don't happen to healthy, fit 59-year-old men. They don't happen to Martin. They don't happen to people I love.

'Come over here to a quiet place', I say and lead Martin to an isolated corner. 'Tell me again'.

'I'm having trouble putting words together'. Martin's voice is more hesitant than usual, slower, although the words are coming out in his normal tones. But he is telling me that it's unusually difficult for him. I know what that means. Something bad is happening in Broca's area of the brain, the area in charge of communicating through language, the region of expressive speech.

Although I am standing perfectly still, I am split frenetically in two. 'This cannot be happening! But it is! Surely it isn't! But it is! Please, please, maybe it isn't?' Suddenly I look up and see my friend Cindy passing by. Cindy is a dear friend and a speech pathologist. I know she will know the same neuropsychology I know.

'Cindy', I call, softly but urgently. She comes over smiling, ready to exchange opinions on the qualities of the dances taught.

'Martin says he's having trouble putting words together'.

She looks at me. I look at her. We both know what we are thinking.

She asks Martin to repeat a couple of tongue-twisting phrases – words he would normally be able to manage with relative ease. He cannot complete them; he is stuck in the middle.

Cindy and I exchange glances again.

'We have to get an ambulance', she says. And I nod. My two selves catch up with each other. We have to get an ambulance.

4

And so it begins.

A few other friends come up, concerned. Word is spreading that something is wrong. We take Martin to a couch so he can lie down. He is not distressed, just puzzled. His colour is normal. His movements are normal. He looks normal. We are becoming the epicentre of a small circle of attention. A part of me is thinking, 'What if this is all about nothing? What if there isn't anything wrong and an ambulance has been called and we end up in a hospital emergency room for no reason? What if I am just making a fuss about nothing and causing such disruption and drama?' People are drifting up, concerned, curious. I hate being the centre of this attention but I need them. I need someone to talk to – someone to confirm the reality of what is happening, someone to ring the ambulance while I stay with Martin, someone just to be there. Cindy tells me she will go to the hospital with me. I nearly cry with gratitude for that gift.

Things begin to happen. Someone says the ambulance men have arrived downstairs and will be up in a few minutes. I collect Martin's parka, backpack, my bags, make sure nothing has been left behind. People drift back to dancing. Everything is so normal except for this one thing that isn't, that cannot, absolutely cannot, be happening. Martin is too young, too fit, too healthy. My mind is skidding and swerving like a crazed rollerblader, swooping on and off the possibility that this could be something serious.

We get downstairs and all the practical, ridiculous trivialities crowd in on me. I get lost two feet outside my front door and here we are in Frankston, needing to follow an ambulance through traffic and unknown streets, to an unfamiliar destination for which I have neglected to get the address. In the best of conditions and with my concentration fully free to focus I will get unnervingly lost. In these conditions, with my mind in a thousand different pieces, I will end up driving in infinite, crazed circles. Cindy, my personal angel, offers to take over the driving while I keep an eye on the ambulance just ahead. The sky is still heavy and the rain has slowed to a trickle as we slowly cruise out of the car park trying to attach invisible towropes to the ambulance just ahead. The conference building slides away and with it all the people improbably dancing. The split in the universe. The one behind us, the one we should have been left in, slipping out of sight.

The ambulance is driving at normal speed. It is not one of those wild rides behind a siren. Cindy has the following and I have the watching under control. As we drive, I suddenly remember the dream I had last week. I recounted it to Martin last Saturday morning, standing in the kitchen and puzzling about it.

It is an odd dream. In it, I am also standing in the kitchen and talking to Martin. Suddenly he freezes mid-sentence, like the freeze-frame of an abruptly halting film. 'Martin…? Martin?' I say. And suddenly he jerks back into motion. 'What happened?' I ask. He shakes his head. 'I got blocked', he says. 'I'm so tired. I got blocked. Nothing could get through'. It is an explanation that makes no sense but, as one does in the dream world, I accept it. Then it happens once more. And again he unfreezes. Then the dream cuts to a scene in Martin's car. I am driving with Cindy to a hospital to get her brain scanned. And there the dream ends.

As I tell Martin about the dream the next morning in the real world, neither of us can figure out where the dream comes from or what it means. Martin is not tired; he is in good health with lots of energy. Cindy, too, is in good health with no reason to go to a hospital, let alone for a brain scan. I don't have brain scans on my mind. Nothing special has happened with either Cindy or Martin to bring them to my dreaming mind. It is a puzzle. Should I tell Cindy about the dream? I wonder to myself. And decide that no, there is no reason to. No one enjoys hearing a dream about themselves where unpleasant things happen. So Martin is the only person I tell it to. Until now. Here I am with Cindy in Martin's car driving to a hospital to get a brain scan. Except that it is Martin's brain that is to be scanned.

'That's weird', says Cindy. 'That's really weird'.

And it is. Seriously weird.

And then suddenly I remember that in my dream, Martin was blocked and froze twice.

'Twice – it couldn't happen twice', I blurt out. 'Why would it happen twice?'

We both shrug and get on with following the ambulance.

The streets wind around totally unfamiliar terrain. Neither of us has a clue where we are. We are just focused on keeping the blocky shape of the ambulance in view. At one point we are separated by traffic lights and we strain our eyes, only letting our breath out when we see that the ambulance has drawn over to the kerb past the lights to wait for us to catch up. Afterwards I will learn that it was Martin who, realising we might lose the ambulance if separated, had the presence of mind to ask the driver to pull up and wait for us.

At last the ambulance draws in to the hospital. Cindy and I maze our way around the car park before finally finding what must be the last parking space left. We exit into drizzle. Martin has been wheeled on ahead of us to the Emergency Department.

A junior doctor appears by Martin's bedside to go through a basic neurological work-up. Martin does well, apart from the hesitancy in his speech and his slowness in finding words. Whatever it is, the effect right now is minor. The doctor is unsure whether it is a TIA (a transient ischaemic attack, or mini-stroke) or the beginnings of a major stroke.

An X-ray is scheduled. If it is a TIA, the symptoms will disappear soon and Martin will be back to normal. It will be a warning sign, needing investigation but not life-threatening today. If it is a stroke, there are larger issues to think about. The first big one is what kind of a stroke – is it one caused by a bleed (a haemorrhagic stroke) or one caused by a clot (an ischaemic stroke)? And if it is a clot, the big question is whether Martin should have clot-busting drugs.

Clot-busting drugs are one of medicine's new magic bullets, designed to dissolve blood clots before they can do further damage. They have a window of opportunity, currently thought to be around five hours. They can be lifesaving and preserve abilities that might otherwise be lost as a result of the stroke. They can also add to bleeding if bleeding has occurred or might occur. In that latter scenario they can be death-dealing, increasing the bleeding and leading to further destruction of brain tissue.

'When exactly did the stroke start?' asks the doctor.

At this point I realise that there are two possible answers. Did it start at 10.30 am, when Martin told me he was stuttering with the cold? Or did it start at 2.00 pm when Martin discovered it was hard for him to find words? If it is the former, the window of opportunity has passed already. If it is the latter, the window of opportunity is open. I know that windows of opportunity must be worked out on averages. This means that for some people, the outliers on the graph, the window of opportunity will be seven hours. What if Martin is an outlier and his window of opportunity is still open, even if the stroke did begin at 10.30 am?

I have told the registrar the story of the stuttering at 10.30 and the difficulty in finding words at 2.00 pm but he is still asking me when the stroke started – he wants to know when I first noticed symptoms. He is asking me to determine the timing. If I tell the doctors that 10.30 am was the beginning, they will close the clot-buster option. On the other hand, what if a bleed is on Martin's horizon? The clot-buster drug will be devastating. I have to make the decision about which time I choose. No one knows which was the true beginning.

The registrars are trying to contact the consultant neurologist to get his opinion. It is a public holiday on a long weekend, so everyone is hard to reach. I go over and over the possibilities in my mind. Which is the best move? Which is the best decision? Martin is taken off for an X-ray and comes back after thirty minutes but it takes hours to find a doctor who can tell me what the scan shows, what is happening. Finally, I catch a registrar. They are sure now that it is not a TIA, that it is the more serious option, a stroke. It has been caused by a clot as there is no bleeding. The clot is very small and so is the area of damage. They are still trying to decide on the clot-buster option. What are the potential negative effects? I ask. It is a powerful drug, comes the answer, and it can be problematic. I am veering towards saying the window is not open for the clot-buster. And then suddenly the consultant calls back.

There is a conversation that comes to me one-sided from my vantage point near the registrar. The consultant decides that the damage is too small and the window too uncertain to warrant the clot-buster. It is a relief to have the decision taken out of my hands. I don't need to flip backwards and forwards over pros and cons I don't fully understand. I can let an expert make a clear, unequivocal decision. It is the first of a series of medical decisions that will need to be made. Its impact – the relief of sitting back and letting the experts tell me what to do – is intense. It has exposed me to the comfort of having someone take over decision-making, but not yet to the dangers of doing that.

Shortly after arriving in hospital, with Martin settled in the Emergency Department bed, I have called our daughter Amantha to let her know what has been happening. Her usual bright answering machine message greets me. I leave my own message, making an effort to sound composed, asking her to ring me as soon as she can. A while later, she still hasn't rung. I leave another one, this time emphasising the 'as soon as you can'. I picture her enjoying the freedom of a long weekend, relaxing with friends – completely unaware that as soon as she answers my call, her world is going to spin itself upside down. By the time she gets my message it is late afternoon. 'Hi Mum', she says breezily, and then, as I tell her what has happened, her voice turns sharp with shock and fear. 'Is he all right? Will he be all right?' I reassure her. It is mild. He is fine. He may only have to stay overnight and then come home. His functioning is good, just a little trouble with words. He is stable. He is calm. He is settled in bed in a ward and he is about to have dinner.

We arrange that Cindy and I will drive home in Martin's car and then Amantha and I will drive back in to Frankston to stay with Martin for the evening. Amantha gets off the phone reluctantly. I can feel the way her life has suddenly jerked off its rails, as mine did a few hours earlier. I realise she is the first person outside the enclosed bubble of the dance group I have talked to. The new reality is leaking out, like a gas dispersing without losing its potency. It is Schrödinger's cat – once observed, its state of being is immutable. And as the news spreads, I have the crazy fantasy that the more people who know, the more irrevocable and real it becomes.

Martin is still bedded down in the Emergency Unit, waiting for his bed in the Stroke Ward to be freed, when Cindy and I say goodbye to him. As we are about to leave, a nurse rustles in to check on him. As she takes his blood pressure and temperature – all normal – she remarks chattily that Martin's new speech hesitancy and the mild blocks he has in finding words will stay with him permanently. She is still going about her business when Cindy and I say goodbye. We go down the elevators, through the corridors, all the way out into the car park with the nurse and her needless, stupid comments on our mind. We have almost reached the car when we simultaneously realise that we cannot leave Martin with those words echoing in the room. When we arrive back at Martin's bed, the nurse has gone and I say firmly and clearly to Martin, 'That nurse has no idea what she's talking about – you're going to recover fully. Your speech is going to be normal again'.

Amantha is waiting for me at home when I arrive with Cindy. Her face is washed-out with apprehension and we hug, the clinging hug of the shocked.

I snap into reassuring mode again and repeat the 'It's small, the effects are mild' mantra. I tell her that all going well, he will be released to come back home in the morning. And even as I say it, I know that 'released' is not the correct terminology. I cannot remember the right word. I can think of the words for going into hospital – 'being admitted' – but for the life of me I cannot think of their opposite. All that comes to mind is 'released to come home', the phrase used for prison inmates, police detainees, the kidnapped, the trapped.

I empty Martin's car of the dance gear we have taken up with us to Frankston – sneakers, dance shoes, spare socks – a pile that looks wildly incongruous as I dump it on the couch. What have these carefree accoutrements got to do with the gut-wrenching grit of the past few hours?

I walk rapidly around the house, trying to collect everything Martin will need for an overnight stay in hospital. The list coalesces and dissipates in my mind as if each object retrieved cancels out another one still waiting – shaver, toothbrush, tooth floss, all the minutiae of daily mindless ritual. Just as I think I have everything, I remember that toothbrush means nothing without toothpaste. And then, just as I am sure I have finally remembered to pack everything, I realise I have forgotten to pack Martin's iPod so that he can listen to his favourite music in hospital. In the middle of a strange and unknown situation, he will be able to close his eyes and be drawn into that other universe of the familiar folk-dance melodies he loves.

Amantha and I drive back to Frankston. Martin has finally been assigned a bed in the Neurology Ward. He is settled in, has eaten dinner and is much as I left him a couple of hours ago. He can speak, although slowly and with some difficulty and fewer words. He can write, stand and walk. Apart from the relatively mild speech difficulty, there are no neurological signs that I can see. The registrar feels the same way. The CT scan came back with nothing major, or even minor, visible. I am starting to feel hopeful.

It is clear that Martin has suffered a minor stroke, but it seems the worst of it is over. If at this stage the damage is mild, indications for a full recovery are excellent. The doctors, though, are still puzzled as to why a fit, healthy man with no predisposing factors should have a stroke out of the blue. They are fixated on this – a mystery that has to be solved. They have asked all the questions but the answers point only to normality.

They keep tugging at these questions of 'why, why, why' – inhabiting as they do a world where there must be an answer for everything. My own past experience of ovarian cancer arriving out of the blue, followed by the recurrence that, statistically speaking, was not supposed to happen, has left me firmly in the 'why not?' camp – a believer in the frivolous irrationality of chance.

As they continue their increasingly frustrated 'whys', the doctors order scans, echocardiograms and blood tests, all the while saying the tests are unlikely to show anything. I find myself experiencing a bemused admiration for their absolute belief that somewhere there will be answers. In that moment, it mystifies me why they cannot understand that sometimes 'shit just happens'. I am grateful for their determination to rule out every possible causative factor, but to myself I am saying, 'This is a blip. It happened for no knowable reason. Martin will recover and it will not happen again. Blips are good. They come and then they go. This is going to clear up. A night in hospital and Martin will be home. We will be normal'.

We leave Martin at around 9.00 in the evening. It is lights-out time and the ward is settling down. Martin seems comfortable, or as comfortable as one can be in these circumstances, and is ready for a night's sleep. I am hopeful that night and rest will work restorative magic in the manner of one of those children's slates that erase dark scribbles with a single swish.

It feels eerily wrong to get home to an empty house. The last time Martin and I spent a night apart was sixteen years ago when I was away at a conference in San Francisco. The house seems strange, dislocated in some way that has nothing to do with geography. Amantha asks me if I would like her to stay overnight. I nod gratefully. The night ahead is going to be long and filled with the possibility of sudden emergency. It is a blessing not to be alone with it.

Amantha goes off to bed. I am exhausted but too wired for sleep. I email some friends to update them on what has happened, do some research on strokes and then drag myself to bed and manage to sleep for a brief two hours. I ring the hospital – it is 2.00 am – to check on Martin. The nurse is reassuring. He is sleeping comfortably and they are checking on him regularly. It feels oddly magical to be so far away in the dark and yet, with the simple act of picking up a phone, to be connected to Martin's distant ward where there is light and motion and people keeping watch through the night.

7 June 2009

I have spent the night phoning the hospital every two hours to check on Martin. With each enquiry, the response is 'No deterioration' and I jelly with relief, but by morning, when I make the 7.00 am call and get the same response, I am uneasily aware of the unsaid other half of the sentence. No deterioration, but no improvement either. I brush my prickling discomfort away – Amantha and I plan to drive in to Frankston at 9.00 am to visit and hopefully bring Martin home. I am imagining that we will take him home, see the required specialists and take it easy as Martin recovers from what now seems to be a minor stroke. It feels manageable. Weird, unnerving, without explanation, but manageable.

At 8.30 am, just before Amantha and I set off, I ring the ward again, to ask them to let Martin know we are on our way.

'How is he?' I ask.

'I'll just go and check', the nurse replies.

She comes back after what seems a longer-than-usual time.

'I'm afraid he's deteriorated. He's just come back from a scan. There's been a bleed'.

The words crack through me with the shock of a high impact collision. It seems insane, to have been ringing every two hours through the night to the same stable message and then suddenly, just as the world has settled down again, to be tipped over into this.

I tell Amantha. We exchange terrified glances, get into the car and drive to whatever is awaiting us in Frankston.

Frankston, normally thirty-one kilometres from Melbourne, has shifted to a distance of a thousand as we drive, desperate to find out what has happened to Martin. Our need to be there 'immediately', 'now', 'at once', is making each kilometre stretch interminably.

The nurse gave no details, simply repeated the mantra that he had 'deteriorated'. 'What does 'deteriorated' mean?' I had asked her. She had merely answered, parrot-like, that I would need to speak to the doctor. And of course there was no doctor around to speak to.

Amantha and I are wound tight, focused on getting there as fast as humanly possible. Focused on the speed limit, when every impulse is telling us to double it. Focused on, and at the same time trying to ward off, the terrible fantasies of what we will see when we do arrive.

Finally, we are at the car park, the hospital and at last in Martin's ward. And there is Martin. Looking just like Martin, until we see that half of his mouth droops as he recognises our presence and attempts a very faint smile of recognition and that he is completely, utterly, absolutely unable to speak. He cannot utter even a single word. He cannot voice a syllable. He cannot make even the most minute sound. It is not emotion that is stopping him from speaking. It is his brain and the neurons, or lack thereof, that the bleed of the 'deterioration' has destroyed.

Plunge, plummet, dive, drop. There are so many words for falling and yet none of them truly conveys the terror of having your feet suddenly, horrifyingly, punched out from under you and no ground to stop your fall. The experience is utterly visceral, as if my body is the first to understand what I am witnessing and my brain's reasoning translator has to struggle for seconds to make sense of why I am feeling this.

Trying to keep my expression calm. I lean forward to kiss Martin. 'Darling, we're here', I say. And then 'How are you feeling?'

Martin shrugs, frustrated, puzzled. He is struggling to talk, visibly trying to force words to come out but there is nothing. No sound at all. Not even coherent movement of his lips.

I tell him what has happened. That he has had a stroke. A mild one that happened yesterday and that this morning there was an extra bleed that has affected his speech. That as the swelling in his brain goes down, he will get better. That the worst is over and that now the healing will begin. That he is going to be okay. The last is not what I believe, but rather the universal croon of mother to hurt child, 'It's going to be okay. It's going to be all right'.

I am telling this to myself as much as to Martin. Even as I speak the soothing words I am desperately searching my memories – back to three decades ago when I did some work with brain-damaged patients at a rehab hospital. I know, of course, that there is a lot of recovery in the weeks and months following a stroke, but 'How much, how much?' is what is screaming through my brain. All I can think of is the parade of patients from those years – certainly recovered from where they were straight after the injury but nowhere near what they used to be. Nowhere near at all.

I get some paper and a biro to see if Martin can communicate by writing. Yesterday afternoon he had no trouble doing this. He takes the pen in his left hand – his right arm is now paralysed, and concentrates. At first I think it is the effort of writing with his non-dominant hand that is holding him up, but then I see that it is not a matter of motor clumsiness – the problem is that he cannot find a way to translate the words in his head into written language. The connections are broken.

I write the letters of the alphabet on a piece of paper to see if he can spell out the words by pointing to them. He looks at the paper baffled. He cannot do this either.

I can see Martin taking in the situation with intense, angry frustration. He knows what words are. He knows what he wants to communicate. Why can he not make the usual effortless connection between thought, word and speech? Why can he not speak the words? Why can he not write them? Why can he not find them when he knows they should be there? He is like a preverbal child in that he simply cannot communicate. He cannot speak words and he cannot write words. He has the advantage over the child in that he understands language. But that advantage, precious as it is, also carries with it the knowledge of what language means and the terrifying fact that he has been stripped of the ability to use it.

I calm Martin down and explain again, briefly, what has happened, reiterating that it will get much better. I add that

Frankston, far away as it is, is a good place to be as it has a specialist Stroke Unit that will be able to give him first-class care. Martin flutters his eyelids in the equivalent of a shrug and settles back down in the bed. Amantha and I find chairs and carry them to the side of Martin's bed. Amantha gets out her laptop to work on; I take out my book in a hopeless attempt to read.

Martin has fallen asleep now, clearly exhausted. The effort of grappling with the after-effects of the stroke, the impact of the swelling and bruising in the brain, is enormously draining – he needs far more sleep than usual. He understands where he is and what has happened but he is fuzzy and groggy, as if thinking for him is the equivalent of someone who has only just learned to walk attempting to run through deep water.

I sit back and for the first time take in our surroundings. Martin is in a four-bed ward in the Neurology Unit. In the bed to his left is a young man, either unconscious or in a medicated sleep. His sister is sitting by his bed, talking to him occasionally, even though he is not responsive. His mother and grandmother are there too. The family is taking shifts to make sure he always has someone with him. Sometimes they talk quietly to each other but mostly they are united in a silence that is emotion concentrated down to its purest essence. The intensity of feeling that radiates from them is as palpable and invisible as a gravitational pull – a tether connecting the young man lying motionless on the bed to the small loving family gathered around him. It has the intensity of Michelangelo's *Pietà*. Every now and then one of their voices becomes audible and the everyday Australian accent forms an odd contrast to the tableau – the ordinariness of our selves and the terrible extraordinariness into which we have been plunged.

The bed opposite Martin's contains another young man who, for the moment, appears to be simply asleep. He is about the same age as the first young man but even in deep sleep he looks different. More alive. More vigorous.

The fourth bed is empty for the moment. This room, for now, is the world.

I go to ask the nurse when the doctors will come by. She shrugs. No one knows. 'Is there a possibility that Martin can see the consultant today?' I ask. That one she does have the answer to. It is a long weekend – the hospital is consultant-free. 'The registrars are in touch with the consultants', she tells me. 'They're keeping track of what's happening'.

Keeping track of is not what I want. I want someone to be there, right here, right now. Someone who knows what they are doing, someone who can tell me what is going on, someone with authority, someone I can trust.

The long weekend means it will be two days before Martin is seen by a consultant, and the horror I feel at such a wait is entirely irrational. There is no current emergency. Martin is stable. He does not need to be rushed into surgery or started on some life-saving medication. The professor's visit on Monday will add nothing new to his treatment, his diagnosis or his prognosis, but I am focusing on it with a maniacal magical-thinking intensity. The professor will tell us what is going on and he will tell us what is going to happen. Embedded in the 'what is going to happen' is the unspoken 'and he will say that Martin is going to get better'.

I sit by Martin's bed, hoping that each footfall brings at least a junior doctor – someone of whom I can ask questions, someone who can tell me more than just the vague wisps of information I have been able to get from the nursing staff. But no one comes.

Finally, a white coat turns into the ward. But not for us. It is the registrar assigned to the young man in the bed on our left. The family members grab him with their eyes as he enters – it is only civilisation that prevents them from grabbing him with their hands. The young doctor goes through a brief examination of his patient – he has obviously been to this bed before. The mother gestures, touches his sleeve.

'When can we see the consultant?' she asks, her voice a monotone of fatigue.

The doctor looks resigned, the faintest tinge of irritation around the edges. 'After the long weekend', he says. And you can hear from his voice that he has said this many times, to many people. 'We're keeping him informed'.

'Please', the mother touches his arm again. 'Please, can you lower the medication? He's so drugged he can't communicate with us. He's not himself. This isn't him. He was better with the other medication'.

'This is what the consultant ordered', the doctor says. 'We have to stick with it'.

'But he doesn't even open his eyes – we can't reach him', says the mother, her hand involuntarily moving to stroke her son's face. 'He's not there. We could talk to him with the other drugs'. She is close to tears.

The young doctor shrugs awkwardly. 'I can't do anything. We have to wait till the consultant sees him'.

'But his consultant won't be here until Tuesday', she says, her voice breaking. 'Tuesday...', her voice trails off with the impossibility of Tuesday.

The doctor shakes his head. 'I can't', he says. 'I can't'.

Martin is dozing on and off. I have my mobile phone with me and it goes off regularly, causing me to jump, work out where the ringing is coming from and then crocodile-wrestle the contents of my bag in an attempt to find it before it stops. I am a techno-moron who has only recently become the owner of a mobile phone. Up till now its purpose has been to reside somewhere in the lower depths of my bag on the off-chance that if I had car trouble away from home I would remember how to use it. The former was more likely than the latter.

My friends texted gaily away and had often offered to teach me. I had once made a half-hearted attempt to learn but ditched it due to the disconcerting way the phone-imp had of anticipating what I wanted to say and saying it wrongly.

Now, sitting and alternately jumping to scrambled attention in Martin's hospital room, I understand for the first time the usefulness of texting. In order to let people know what is happening, I have to ring them. If they are not in, I have to leave messages. They ring back, invariably when I cannot talk, and then I have to ring them back again. And again. And I have to do it all one call at a time, one person at a time, one message at a time, over and over again. Texting is the answer to this constant tag-game of missed connections. If only I had paid more attention.

I also don't want to discuss Martin's condition in front of Martin, so once I have finally located the ringing phone I then have to exit the ward to convey the news. I don't want to turn my phone off because, of course, I don't know how to retrieve messages. So I jump, scramble, run and return at regular intervals during the day.

The morning has passed with still no sighting of a doctor. Martin is drowsy and asleep for much of the time. In his waking moments he seems oddly calm – perhaps inert is the better word. I ask him how he is feeling in a kind of twenty-questions parody – Are you anxious? Upset? Depressed? To all of these he shakes his head. In between talking to him, I sit by his bed and attempt to read, although only three pages of my book will have actually been turned by the end of the day.

I unwrap a sandwich from our stash of provisions, which consists of boiled eggs and cheese sandwiches, but give up after one bite. My appetite has lit out for the hills. It doesn't happen often in my life but when it does, I am struck all over again by the fact that it is not the food that contains the flavour, labour as some of us might over the intricacies of spices and cuisine, it is our brain. If whatever determines taste-pleasure in the brain is switched off, a thousand *MasterChef* contestants cannot switch it back on again

Martin is being given fluids intravenously. As the lunchtime trays with their tinny music jolt their way around the ward, I see that Martin has no lunch tray scheduled. The nurse nods when I ask her about this. 'We have to check his swallowing', she says.

'Swallowing?' I ask. This is the first time I have heard this mentioned.

'He can't swallow because of the stroke, so if he were to eat or drink, he could choke'.

has caused a great deal more damage than yesterday's event, which is like a pinprick in comparison. The registrar doesn't know how much function Martin will recover, but the gloominess of his delivery suggests he is not optimistic. We will simply have to wait and see, he says. Right now the brain is bruised and swollen as well as damaged by the stroke, and as the swelling goes down in the next few weeks there will be some recovery. The brain cells which have had their oxygen cut off are already dead. They will not recover, he says and the damaged area is large. I can see Martin's expression of horror as he hears the doctor say this.

As soon as the registrar leaves the room, I go to Martin's side. 'Forget about what he said', I tell Martin. 'The brain is much more plastic than people used to think it was. It can relearn skills, find new circuits and even grow new neurons. This research is new – a lot of doctors aren't up with it yet. There are things you can do that will make a big difference. You'll get back your abilities. You'll be able to speak again. You'll be able to write and use your right hand again. I'll tell you what to do and how to do it and we'll be able to get there'.

I do indeed know that there has been some revolutionary recent research on brain plasticity, but it is not my specialist area and, in truth, I don't know how much ability Martin can get back. But I know that the research suggests there is more room for improvement than the doctor thinks. And I know, too, that it will require steady determined work on Martin's part, and how much better it is to do that work in an optimistic frame of mind than in the pessimistic one the doctor's words suggest.

Martin nods as I tell him these things. He understands and he believes me. It settles him a bit.

Up until now Amantha and I have been communicating with Martin through a protracted form of twenty questions. We ask and he shakes his head or nods. When nursing or medical staff come in, asking questions to do with topics such as Martin's medical history, allergies and so on – any questions that require more than a yes or a no – the conversation is routed through me. When it is us who want the information, the process is relatively easy – simply formulate a question that can be answered with a nod, a shake or a one-shouldered shrug. When it is Martin who wants to ask or tell us something, the process is harder – more akin to a tricky game of charades at an inebriated party with the rules insisting that the charade be enacted while semi-recumbent and with very limited movement.

I will be with Martin from 9.00 am until 8.30 pm each day. I am lucky in that I run my own private practice and can take time off or shift work hours if I need to. During the time that I am with Martin, I can deal with communicating whatever needs to be communicated to staff. What happens, though, when I am not there and Martin wants something? He has the standard nurses' call button by his bed, but if he presses it and they come, how can he let them know what he wants?

I find a piece of paper and write in bold letters as many things as I can think of: TOILET, PAIN, MEDICATION, TOO COLD, TOO HOT, SHOWER, UNCOMFORTABLE. The list is appallingly short. 'Hungry' and 'thirsty' obviously don't come into it when one is on nil orally, but I am sure I have left out realms of words, requests and communications. This brief list seems ridiculous as a summary of all one's needs, but I check with Martin to see if that covers everything and he nods.

As the ward begins its bedding-down preparations at 8.30 pm, Amantha and I reluctantly leave. In this age of super-communication, it is eerie to know that even though we are both accessible by phone, I will not be able to communicate with him until tomorrow morning when I am by his bedside again. Without a voice and without written language, there is nothing he can tell me until we are face to face. And of course even then, what he can tell me is limited.

Amantha and I drive home still fogged with shock. I am making a list internally of all the things I need to do that might be helpful for Martin. I will make him a hypnosis tape tonight that he can play on his iPod in hospital. It will help him relax and feel calmer and more positive. It could also bring down his cortisol levels, which could in turn help his body and brain in their recovery. Within the tape, I will also get him to imagine speaking and moving his arm and leg, which might help activate neural circuits in his brain. Research has shown that when you imagine playing tennis, for example, while in a hypnotic trance, the appropriate motor neurons you would use to perform that action fire in the brain. It might help and it cannot hurt. And I have a lot of research to do.

I remember a Finnish study I recently came across which showed that listening to two hours of music of any genre post-stroke resulted in significant improvement in the areas of verbal memory, focused attention and other cognitive abilities. In addition, the 'music' patients were less depressed and their mood was less confused. The researchers compared the music-listening group to both a neutral control group and a group who listened to spoken-word recordings. The music group did far better than either of the other two groups. That's an easy intervention to organise for Martin. He loves his music and is already playing it on the iPod Amantha and I brought in for him last night. If I can put together as many as I can of these research-based interventions, even though individually they might only make a small difference, perhaps taken together they can amount to a large difference for Martin's recovery.

It is late evening when we get home, and the pitch-darkness of the house feels like a presence that in a film would require ominous background music. I race around irrationally switching on all the lights that I can.

Amantha and her partner Shannon prepare dinner. The possibility of eating still seems to me to rate somewhere just above the likelihood of my taking up skydiving for fun. It occurs to me that there must be a diet book in here somewhere – The Stroke Survivor's Spouse's Diet?

I go upstairs to send email updates about Martin and to reclaim two books that have been waiting on my bookshelf, unbeknown to me, for this day – *My Stroke of Insight* by Jill Bolte Taylor and *The Brain That Changes Itself* by Norman Doidge. I find them – a semi-miraculous experience – among my thousands of randomly shelved books, and then spend some time at the computer googling research.

Neuropsychology is not my area of speciality but I am fortunate in that I know enough of it to be able to research and understand the latest findings and think about how to apply them to Martin's situation. My training as a psychologist also enables me to evaluate the research and articles available on the web critically. It is essential to be able to do this, as information on the web varies from serious, solid research to proclamations that would make any scientist's hair stand on end and are either useless or in worst cases damaging. I read through several articles on stroke and make notes about what I should put in Martin's hypnosis tape.

After making the tape, I head to the kitchen to boil eggs for tomorrow's mobile food needs. Amantha and Shannon are asleep in the new makeshift bedroom at the end of the house. Amantha, who runs her own business, has been able to cancel her appointments and will sleep over for the next few days. I take some paracetamol for my aching back and crawl into bed.

I wake two hours later into the post-midnight house. I am covered in sweat and shivering violently. I ring the hospital to see how Martin is doing. He has been very agitated, the nurse says, but is now back asleep. I go back to bed but sleeping is clearly not on the agenda for me. I wrap myself up in layers, topped by my old woollen dressing gown – the freezing cold of the unheated night-time house feels too much like the freezing cold of fear. If I can ward it off, away from my body, perhaps I can keep it away from my heart.

I go upstairs to send a few update emails to friends I have not been able to contact during the day. Faith (not her real name), my dearest friend of thirty years, is overseas at a psychoanalytic conference. We would normally speak to each other at least once a week and have supported each other through all the various crises in our lives in the caring, steadfast way of the best families. We feel like family even though we have no bloodlines in common and were brought up on different continents. We have been there for each other through all those decades in both tough times and fair. If I have a dream that is puzzling me or an emotional issue I want to explore, Faith is the friend I turn to — and the same holds for her. We trust each other's knowledge of our deepest selves. It is Faith to whom I most wish I could talk right now. I write telling her what has happened, and even the experience of writing feels as if I am speaking to her.

I spend the rest of the night reading *The Brain That Changes Itself* and related research, all the while thinking about practical implementations. Every two hours, I ring the hospital to see how Martin is doing. One end of the seesaw upon which Martin's future is precariously, exquisitely, balanced holds the hopeful possibility of improvement, but the other end is weighted by the possibility of more strokes, further damage. Right now, each end is in perfect balance — no improvement, no deterioration. In this night, everything feels dependent upon a feather.

Martin's brain has, in medical terms, suffered a massive insult. It is a phrase that creates the endearing image of the insulted one rearing back with 'How could you say such a thing?' indignation. In medical reality, insult simply and plainly means damage. A massive insult has nothing to do with words or feelings, it is about terrible, destructive physical damage. Neurons in the speech area of Martin's brain, where the bleeding has occurred, have been deprived of oxygen for too long, they are dead. The scale of the damage is extensive but we will not know the exact extent until the swelling goes down. There has been universal pessimism from the doctors about how much function will come back and whether Martin will be able to speak again, let alone speak fluently and recover what we take so thoughtlessly for granted — the ability to communicate thoughts, wishes, needs.

It is only somewhere towards dawn, as I am sitting at the computer, straining to decipher the research language of neurotransmitters and neurophysiology, that I am suddenly felled by the realisation that if I had picked the later of the start times for Martin's stroke – if Martin had not mentioned that he was stuttering with cold four hours before he told me he was having trouble finding words, and the clot-buster drug had been administered on the basis of that, Martin might not now be alive. The clot-buster drugs have a side effect of making bleeding harder to control. With that in his system, Martin's secondary bleed might have gone on to become an unstoppable haemorrhage.

8 June 2009

This morning, with all the intellectual acuity of someone who has had two hours' sleep for each of the past two nights, I am gripped by the idea that singing a song before we set out on the road to Frankston will help keep our spirits up. I suspect I am motivated by images of Dorothy, Scarecrow, Lion and Tin Man singing as they set out along the yellow brick road to Oz. In keeping with musical theatre tradition, I pick 'The Sun'll Come Out Tomorrow' from *Annie* and print out the words. Amantha and Shannon are not so convinced that a singalong will raise our spirits but reluctantly comply. My efforts to stir up musical spirits on successive mornings, however, are politely but firmly declined. The road to Frankston remains, as always, interminably long. Definitely not yellow brick and definitely not leading to the wizard.

Martin barely smiles as we come in. He is looking twenty years older, pale and fragile. I kiss and hug him in greeting and go through the usual twenty questions routine to ask how he is feeling.

'Are you in pain?'

Shake of the head.

'Are you sad?'

Shake of the head.

'Are you frightened?'

Shake of the head.

'Are you frustrated?'

Violent nodding.

I show him the hypnosis tape I have made him. He has used hypnosis several times before and knows how well it works. He has asked me to make him tapes on several occasions in the past. I tell him it is part of what will help him recover and that he should play it several times a day.

The doctors have not done their rounds yet so I go in search of the nurses for information. Martin's condition remains unchanged, I am told. He still cannot make a sound or swallow, and the right-side paralysis of his arm is still as it was yesterday – no movement at all. When I look at him, however, his smile seems a tad less crooked and he can now close his right eyelid properly. 'Good signs, good signs', I repeat to myself, as if the words themselves are a form of magic.

I sit by Martin's bed holding his hand. He has his eyes closed. Not asleep, not awake. In the bed to our left, the unconscious young man seems much the same as he was yesterday. His family have been sitting with him in rosters. This morning his sister is in with him. Like her brother, she is young – late teens, maybe early twenties. She talks to him softly, strokes his hair, massages his feet, all so calmly and lovingly that I want to go over and hug her. Her grandmother comes in later to join her. They sit together quietly, totally present for the young man they love.

Martin has been alternately drowsing and listening to music on his iPod. I chat to him, telling him what has been happening, thinking of small things that might make him smile. I tell him a little about the research I have been reading and how plastic the brain is and that he is going to get better. On one occasion, a funny anecdote I have been relaying raises a smile and I can see for the first time that it is nearly a proper smile, not like the crooked semiparalysed half-smile of his first day. I light up as if I have won Lotto. 'You're smiling properly', I say. 'It's fantastic – the healing's beginning!' Martin smiles wanly and it is true – his smile is better.

I leave the ward to tell Amantha, who is working on her laptop in another room. As I pass the young man's bed, his grandmother leans towards me and says, 'It's good to see you smile'.

'Thank you', I say, nearly in tears at the small kindnesses of people in the grip of their own terror.

When I come back, I take a box of chocolate left by one of our visitors over to the family as a gift.

'Thank you', they say in turn, and we touch each other's shoulders, knowing what we are really thanking each other for is the rare, sweet gift of witnessing each other. Of truly seeing each other's pain and saying in what small way we can, 'I am there. I see'. From now on, we will say hello and goodbye to each other whenever we come and go, brief greetings that contain a library of words within them.

A nurse arrives to check on Martin's vitals. This is the nurse who specialises in running gags infused with a schtick any stand-up comedian would be proud of. She ribs Martin good-naturedly and he responds by smiling. She is a marvel. Her compatriot, the other nurse who also takes care of our section of the ward, is equally marvellous – always smiling, gentle and ready to go the extra mile for her patients' comfort. The quality of these two spirits among the drabness, the physical disintegration that comes with neurological damage, the messes, indignities and psychic horror of the ward, is as startling and refreshing as tropical flowers in winter.

And we have seen a lot of these two nurses over the last couple of days, the main reason being that patient number three, the young man in the bed opposite us, who looked as if he was sleeping off the effects of a hard party, has woken up. And in a triumph of intuitive medical diagnosis, it turns out that he was, indeed, sleeping off the effects of a hard party. Whatever drugs he was using have left their mark. He is uncoordinated, uninhibited and determined to do the opposite of everything the doctors and nurses tell him to do. He is not supposed to get out of bed as his lack of balance makes him a danger to himself. He is supposed to stay in overnight so they can monitor him until the party drugs wear off. Every five minutes he lurches out of bed to get dressed and check himself out so he can go home. Every five minutes an overworked nurse has to rush in, get him back into bed and explain to him again that he is to stay overnight. This performance continues throughout the morning, ceasing only when someone assigns one of the nurses to sit by his bed for the afternoon, deeming it the only method of ensuring that the young man remains in it.

This is the young man's third such admission to the ward this year. He clearly has the hospital filed in the same category as hangover cures. Go out partying, get hammered, get drugged, go to the hospital, get cleared and do it all over again. I look at the terribly ill patients in this ward – here through severe illness or accident, all in desperate need of the nurses who would still be overworked even if staff numbers were doubled. And then I look at the one nurse assigned to spend her precious time sitting by the bed of this idiot (I have cast all political correctness aside), and my blood boils. As I walk out into the corridor, I catch another nurse raising her eyebrows and shaking her head in wonderment at the monumental load this young man is placing on the ward. 'There should be a "three-strikes and you're out" rule for people like him', I say in Attila the Hun mode. 'The third time you do this in a year, you should be patched up in emergency and turfed out'. The nurse nods in vigorous agreement.

A few friends have been dropping in to see Martin. The visits are necessarily brief but he lights up with them, particularly those friends who come with light-hearted hospital jokes and humour. His mood lifts when they come and drops when they leave.

One of his visitors is Denise, our close friend and dance teacher. After she has greeted Martin, she leans over and whispers something in his ear. Martin nods in response. Denise looks relieved. I do not have to be a lip-reader to know what was just said. Denise knows how passionate Martin is about his dancing. He has been dancing for four years now, knows 300 dances and is planning on adding an extra zero to that number. Denise has just asked Martin whether he still remembers the sequences of his favourite dances and Martin has said yes.

I had been dancing for two years when my regularly repeated 'Why don't you try it, you'll like it?' finally led Martin to his first class. Within four weeks he was addicted, both to the music and the choreography. Israeli folk-dance music ranges from soulfully lyrical to joyously wild, the tempos from slow waltz to jitterbug-fast. Each dance has a fixed and unique sequence of steps and is danced to one particular song. There are more than 3,000 songs and dances in existence and the number is constantly growing. Martin is in love. He spends all his time learning new dances and notating them on his website. The music, courtesy of his iPod, accompanies him wherever he goes. With his slim build and grace on the dance floor, he is becoming the Fred Astaire of the local scene. And even now, when he can no longer access expressive verbal language, Martin can still remember the language of dance.

I am just realising that I have read the same page of my book six times over when the herd-like sound of multiple trampling feet comes echoing down the corridor. In the old American West, this would mean buffalo. In the hospital, it means consultant. The extra footsteps signify the team, trailing comet-tail fashion in his wake.

There is a moment of held breath while I wait to see if it is our bed he is headed for. He passes the first bed without looking, consults some notes in his hand and yes, his destination is us. This is the professor who was consulted by phone on what seems years ago, that Saturday afternoon when Martin was admitted.

There are introductory handshakes all around and I go through the history of what has happened. The prof is still trying to find the elusive 'why' of the stroke. I go through Martin's family history and his own medical history. There is nothing to indicate any risk of stroke.

'Has he had any recent surgeries?'

'He had a laser procedure for a benign, enlarged prostate in February, four months ago', I say.

The prof shakes his head. 'That's too far away to have any influence'. He is obviously wondering about anything that could have induced blood clots that might have travelled to the brain. He asks a couple more questions, the answers to which are all negative. Nothing in Martin's history or presentation is throwing up any clues.

And then, the prof asks one more question – one I have not heard before. 'What is your goal?' he says to Martin.

As Martin's answering service, I am struck slightly dumb for a second in the face of so many glaringly obvious answers – to speak, to walk, to use his right hand, to get out of this place. But it is obvious from the enquiring and expectant looks on the multiple faces of the team that this is not what they are after. What they want is a Goal – the kind that can be put on motivational posters and cunningly placed above workstations.

'I'm sure I can answer that', I say smoothly. 'Martin would like to get back to dancing again'. The team smile. I have answered correctly. Martin also smiles – that is exactly what he wants to do.

The prof says, 'That's a good goal to work towards'.

I nod too, but inside me a voice is wailing, 'What about to swallow, what about to say a few words, what about to go to the toilet by himself?' Dancing, in the complicated rhythms and sequences we have been used to, seems about as achievable as attempting to fly by way of leaping into the air Superman style.

The prof now gets down to the serious work of the neurological examination. He tests whether Martin can follow a moving finger with his eyes. He points to pictures to see if Martin can identify the matching words. He asks Martin to raise his leg as high as he can and resist the prof's pressure to bring it down. He asks him to point his tongue in various directions and gives Martin a range of other tests and activities designed to gauge the level of damage to his brain. At one point I realise that Martin, a brilliant computer analyst, has lost the ability to count above the number five. At another point, as the prof tells Martin to do one thing, Martin keeps repeating his response to the previous task. The prof turns to me.

'Perseveration', he says.

'No', I respond too promptly, too automatically. 'It's just that the tasks are coming too fast. He's still processing them'. That is true. I am sure it is true.

The prof shakes his head.

Perseveration, the tendency to get stuck, broken-record style, repeating one action or phrase, is a classic sign of brain damage. I have seen it a hundred times in patients. It is impossible that I am seeing it now in Martin.

The examination proceeds. With every second, the extent of Martin's deficits is becoming horrifyingly clear. The prof finishes and recaps his findings: Martin has suffered extensive damage to the left frontal lobe, centring around Broca's area – the area concerned with the production of speech. The area controlling the right arm is very close to Broca's, which is why Martin's arm is paralysed, and there is a similar reason for the weakness in his right leg. He underlines the fact that the return of swallowing is essential in order for Martin to avoid having a nasogastric tube inserted, and equally essential in order for him to be moved on to a rehabilitation hospital. This ward is intended for acute patients in need of medical treatment and care. The professor closes by saying there is hope that Martin will regain some of his functioning with time. From his expression, it is clear that the subtext of 'some' is 'a little' and that of 'hope' is 'if we keep our fingers crossed'. I look at Martin's face as the prof pronounces this and hope he is not reading the subtext as clearly as I am.

He displays the pictures of Martin's CT scans. The initial one, taken on the Saturday, when he was first admitted, shows nothing – the damage is so small it is invisible. The CT scan from Sunday morning, however, displays a shockingly large black area the size of a golf ball – this is the subsequent bleed, measuring three by three by three centimetres in the left-hemisphere speech area.

As soon as the doctors have exited, I go over to Martin's bedside and repeat my mantra: 'Ignore what they say. They haven't worked with the latest research – it's too new for them. The brain is much more capable of repair than they think. You're going to be using all the new techniques and research they haven't tried out. You're going to surprise them. You're going to get better'.

Martin subsides into sleep – the prof's visit has left him exhausted. I try desperately, as usual, to make myself believe what I have said.

An hour later, a young woman enters the room. The speech pathologist has come in for her first visit. I watch her put Martin through his paces, of which of course there are very few. She has sheets of exercises that look as if they have come out of a first-grade primer: pages of pictures with matching words on the opposite pages, words in large print with letters missing, simple one-syllable words waiting to be pronounced out loud. It is the kind of worksheet the average seven-year-old is bored with. For Martin they might as well be postdoctoral quantum mechanics equations.

Martin can recognise words that are written and spoken, but he cannot write them, cannot formulate the required sequences of letters that make up words, cannot even point to appropriate letters. He has no way of expressing his inner comprehension of spoken and written language – he is still unable to make even a sound, let alone pronounce a word. The speech pathologist assures Martin that as the swelling in his brain goes down, things will get easier. She will come back tomorrow and also test his swallowing again. Before she goes, she leaves us with a treasure: a sheet of paper with pictures and words of all the basic things Martin might want to communicate to staff or visitors – the professional, expanded version of the communications sheet I made up for Martin the day before.

As we drive home that night, I am again thankful for Amantha's presence and also for her willingness to drive us in and out. I have had a bad back for a few years – short spurts of driving are enough to aggravate it – and I cannot imagine what the hour of driving to Frankston would do to it. As I think this, I remember that just three days ago, that bad back and the exhaustion of being well and truly run-down were at the top of my yearning-to-solve problem list. Now, although my back is aching with the nagging thoroughness of a sit-com mother-in-law, I am barely thinking about it.

Decades ago I bought a greeting card I still have tucked away somewhere in the depths of an old filing cabinet. The front of the card shows a little cartoon character looking hopefully upwards. The caption above it says, 'You are the answer to my prayers'.

When the card is flipped open, the same cartoon character appears, puzzlement now mingled with his hopefulness. The caption reads, 'You're not what I prayed for exactly, but apparently you're the answer'. Martin's stroke, it appears, is the antidote I hadn't exactly asked for to the problem of ruminating about bad backs and fatigue. Not the answer to the bad back and fatigue, just the answer to the problem of thinking about them.

Back home, I have to start looking for some of the essential paperwork that accompanies an experience like this – the insurance policy that you buy, planning never to use. I know Martin has both life insurance and income-protection insurance, covering illness that stops him from working. It is the income-protection insurance I am looking for, but despite the marvellous neatness of Martin's files, I cannot see it anywhere. I try several places but it has vanished. And it is too late to ring the insurance agent. I write it on the long list for tomorrow's tasks and get on to the job of emailing updates to friends, researching and pyjama-washing that now form the odd triumvirate of my regular evening activities.

Again, I fall into bed at 12.00 and am up again at 2.00 am. No sleep. But plenty of time for research, with my computer screen occasionally being put on hold while I make the two-hourly phone calls to Martin's ward to check on his night. The report is uniformly 'No deterioration'. I have learned to be thankful for that.

9 June 2009

By morning, my brain is feeling like grated cheese and my body slightly worse. I pack the standard boiled eggs and sandwiches, consider but discard the impulse to promote another singalong of 'Tomorrow' and heave myself into the car with Amantha for the interminable drive to Frankston. As we drive, I will myself to be energised and cheerful. It will do Martin no good to see me drag myself in looking exhausted.

As we enter the ward Martin is lying in his bed, not yet aware of our presence, tears oozing down his cheeks. My breath catches. I stroke his hand and he calms down after a few moments.

controlled, even overly rational person, not given to great highs or lows. What if this is who Martin is now – at the mercy of the rages, the poor impulse control and the shocking irrational volatility that brain damage often brings?

I calm myself down and go back into the ward. Martin seems sheepish, as if he has had some realisation of how far he went. And it is then that I realise the other thing that happened during his outburst – he made a sound. That guttural growl of rage is the first sound he has made in two days. A breakthrough!

'You made a sound. Your first sound!' I hug him with the excitement of a football fan witnessing the match-winning goal.

Martin is not as excited. I can see that for him a sound is such a minuscule achievement in the face of what he has lost that it is nothing.

'It's the beginning', I say. 'It means things are starting to work again. It will only get better from now on. You'll be able to speak again'. And as always, I am willing myself to believe the words I speak.

Martin offers a small smile – I note with relief that it is still nearly symmetrical. And the hours crawl on.

At noon, the day is broken by an unexpected visit from Cindy and her husband John. After they have said hello to Martin, Cindy urges me to come down to the cafeteria and have lunch with them. It seems like an astonishing suggestion, and I realise I have moved so far from the normal routines and delineations of a day that the idea of eating lunch in a cafeteria with friends seems unthinkably exotic and strange.

It is unbelievably wonderful to sit for an hour in face-to-face conversation with caring friends. For the last couple of days, I have had a job to do with all the people I have been in contact with. With Amantha and Martin, my focus has been to protect them; with the medical staff, my job has been to ask the right questions, check what they are doing and extract the information I need in order to help Martin. It is so nourishing to sit with Cindy and John and simply talk about what has been happening.

And being face to face makes so much difference. I have spoken to friends on the phone and it has been good and comforting, but nothing has prepared me for the difference a physical presence actually makes. It is like the difference between thin broth and rich chunky soup. It is my first visceral experience of what we have lost in the days of texts, emails and mobile phone calls on the run.

I feel refreshed when I go back upstairs to Martin. He has quietened, and thankfully that outburst of unnerving rage is never repeated.

Up until now Martin has been unwilling to play his hypnosis tape and reluctant to do the exercises the physio left for him. It is utterly understandable in the overwhelmed state he is in, but I decide that it is now time to step in as coach. I press him to play the hypnosis tape and he agrees, in part I think in contrition for his previous outburst. I settle him down with the tape and he is noticeably calmer when it is finished. Amantha helps him with the physio exercises. It feels good to be doing something, both for him and for ourselves.

At some point in the afternoon I remember to ask Martin about his income protection insurance. He shakes his head at me. 'Do you know where it is?' I ask again. His headshake is more vehement this time, with the intensity of someone trying to say more than no.

I tilt my head, trying to understand what he means. He shakes his head again, trying to make his body say the words.

'You have got income insurance?' I finally ask. It is impossible that he has not. I can remember when we decided to buy it, years ago. I got a cheap one for me but Martin bought a first-class one from the insurance broker and we have had it ever since.

But Martin is shaking his head again. He is emphatic.

He doesn't have income insurance. He must have cancelled it without telling me. The cold knowledge unnerves me. All the mental maths and calculations I have been doing over the past couple of days – the costs of private rehab hospitals with their private rehab specialists – physiotherapists, speech therapists, have involved income insurance. I will have to start again.

The afternoon passes slowly. The ward exists in its own time in the way of islands, not ruled by the clock but rather by arrivals and departures. The consultant with his gaggle of students, the tea trolleys, the assorted allied health therapists and, more rarely, the changeover of occupants.

The young man in the bed next door is still there, seemingly unchanged through these last few days. The partygoer has finally gone, to the relief of patients, staff and anyone else he may have encountered. His place has been taken by an elderly man whose wife sits beside him with the white-faced, sightless stare of someone unwoken from a nightmare.

Just before dusk, a nurse arrives with a small container of liquid. We tense again. Is Martin still able to swallow? He takes the container in his good left hand and raises it to his lips. The world stops. And he swallows. Elation takes over for this small moment of the day.

As usual it is well after dark when we get home. Friends have been generously leaving food for us and we are touched. It is such a practical and caring gesture at a time when there is no space to cook.

I get to bed and am astonished and grateful to wake after four hours sleep instead of the two hours I have become accustomed to over the last few nights. I feel ridiculously energised by having an amount of sleep that in a previous life I would have been bemoaning bitterly. 'Four hours feels *so* much better than two', I say in amazement to a friend. The puzzled silence that follows tells me that no, she has not been there, done that.

10 June 2009

As we watch in excitement, Martin's drip is taken out – he can swallow well enough to drink and eat for himself. The professor sails into the ward and his smile takes in the absence of drip. He goes through the usual neuro checklist – the differences are tiny but there. And most important is the swallowing. Martin can go to rehab, he pronounces. We have graduated, not summa cum laude, but at least we have graduated. We are on to the next stage.

I have been hoping all this time that the next stage is not going to involve Frankston. I have been frantically researching rehab options and am being universally told that the speech therapy and physiotherapy departments at South-Central Rehabilitation Hospital are first class. And South-Central Rehab is close to us – we are in its catchment area. In addition it is a public hospital, which means that the huge costs of private rehabilitation will not be an issue. A transfer to South-Central becomes my new North Star.

A nurse arrives at Martin's bedside in the afternoon with the 'glad tidings' expression on her face. We lean forward expectantly. 'Martin's well enough to be transferred to a rehab hospital', she says excitedly. 'He's being transferred to Aberdon'.

'Aberdon Rehabilitation Hospital', she says, in deference to our blank looks. 'It's just a few minutes from here'.

And an hour away from home.

'It's very comfortable', she continues, as my spirits drop, 'luxurious compared to this. Martin will have his own room and rehab specialists on tap'.

The last phrase cheers me up a little. While I work to get Martin to South-Central, at least he will have hot and cold running speechies and physios. That's the most important thing.

A couple of hours later, the transfer, involving ambulances, complicated directions and shadowing techniques worthy of any 'Follow that taxi' spy story begins. Eventually, after traffic and terrain that require high-level weaving skills, we arrive at Aberdon. It is hotel-like in comparison to the cramped and crowded wards of Frankston Hospital. Martin not only has his own room, he has his own en suite. The assigned greeter shows us the layout and says all patients are required to dress in street clothes during the day and to come down to meals in the dining room.

It is now late afternoon so Martin will be in time for dinner. It is reassuring to see Martin's comfortable accommodation and to know he is in an after-care hospital specially designed for his needs.

Amantha and I decide we will leave at dinnertime (family are not encouraged to eat with patients) and for the first time since this began will have an evening not spent in hospital.

I unpack Martin's bag and toiletries and he points to what he wants to wear. His right leg is still very weak and I am trying to help him get his trousers on, but he is wildly impatient and pushes me away so he can do it himself. Before I can react he has stood up, tangled himself up in the trousers and fallen. And hit his head on the cupboard.

I help Martin sit up. He is not bleeding, he has not lost consciousness, he is not dizzy. He signals that he is okay. A nurse comes rushing in and I explain that Martin has just tripped and knocked his head a little against the cupboard. She moves into high-action mode. Other nurses are called. A medico. There are no extra neurological signs present but Martin will have to be monitored constantly throughout the evening in case the knock to his head has started any bleeding from the area of stroke damage in his brain. There are discussions about whether to transport him back to Frankston Hospital for another CT scan.

The doctor eventually makes the decision to wait and watch. Amantha and I also settle down for the evening of watching and waiting. Finally, at the patients' lights-out time, we leave. I wake through the night to check on Martin's progress. I cannot believe that a minute's thoughtless impulse could threaten his whole recovery, and I alternately steam with fury and shiver with fear.

11 June 2009

This morning I read Martin the riot act — he has to be careful, he has to be patient and he has to accept help. He nods sheepishly and we hug. The Aberdon morning starts.

To be precise, the Aberdon morning is supposed to start. It starts all right, in the astrophysical sense of things: the sun rises, the darkness departs, and so on. But the stream of busy allied health professionals I have anticipated does not show. I go to enquire at the desk as to when the physio, the speech pathologist, the occupational therapist and the consultant will be arriving to set the rehabilitation in motion. I get a blank look for an answer.

I settle down with Martin to wait. Surely it's just a small delay. At Frankston Hospital we were told how good it would be to be transferred to a rehab hospital where they could really get to grips with helping Martin.

Time passes. Getting to grips seems to be the last thing on the mind of the assorted allied health staff. They have not even worked up to limp handshakes or air kisses. Martin remains unvisited by anyone but the tea lady. By late afternoon my patience is wearing thin. I collar a physio strolling past.

'My husband is recovering from a stroke and needs to have his rehab program started', I say. 'His arm is completely paralysed'.

The physio stares at me disdainfully. 'Physios only work with the lower half of the body'.

And before I can even snort with disbelief, he has vanished. I go down to the desk. 'I need to see Martin's rehab consultant'.

The receptionist looks up from her doodles. 'She's not here'.

'Well when she gets here, I'd like to see her'.

The receptionist gives an 'in your dreams' roll of her eyes.

I simmer back to Martin's room. Amantha and I will have to fill in for the missing therapists. I write some simple words on paper – pairs of objects that go together – salt and pepper for instance, and see whether Martin can match them. These familiar pairings of words – bread and butter, cart and horse – are so ingrained in our speech memories that they are usually easier to retrieve than other words that don't have the automatic connections these pairings have. Martin tries his best but is no more successful than yesterday. When I have finished, Amantha takes Martin through some of the exercises the physio at Frankston Hospital went through with him. Again, there is seemingly no change.

By the end of the day our amateur efforts have still been the only visible attempts at therapy, but we have no speech material to work with. Picture books. First-word books. These are the things we need. We manage to make it to Southland shopping mall in the hour before closing and launch into a sped-up version of mall-aerobics. We race frantically through bookshop after bookshop, trying to find children's books with simple kindergarten words and matching pictures that we can use to improvise therapy. It seems urgent that we start the process of exercising Martin's brain, encouraging it to rebuild and reconnect its resources. Shelf after shelf leaves us still without a single book. The children's books available here are pitched at a higher level of written and verbal comprehension than Martin is currently capable of – a chilling thought. Finally we snaffle two books – each at either end of the very long shopping mall – that scrape through with at least some of my list of requirements. They will have to do.

At home, I turn to the now familiar routine of boiling eggs and making sandwiches for our lunch tomorrow. Martin has requested a longer hypnosis tape – a good sign – so I settle down to make that. And then upstairs to the computer, for both more research and to email updates on Martin's condition to friends.

Because I am in hospital with Martin from dawn till dusk, there is no chance to see friends. Short phone calls and emails are the only contact I have. Friends ring every day, and even though our contact is usually brief and burdened by the static of Aberdon's aversion to telecom network frequencies, the fact that they are thinking of us and holding us in their hearts is enormously comforting. And each evening, no matter how late, I sit down, in what has now become a ritual, and 'talk' into the computer, sending update emails and more personal ones to special friends.

Faith is still overseas but is writing loving notes to me – each feeling like a virtual hug from across the oceans. And a hug is what I long for. It is something that phone calls and emails, no matter how caring, cannot give – the sheer visceral comfort of being enveloped in a friend's loving arms. She has had trouble getting through by phone but can email. And even though she is thousands of miles away, I feel comforted in the knowledge of being cared for.

That sense, of being cared about, is the most powerful elixir. Study after study shows that patients who have good friendship and family networks do better than those who don't. I have always understood this intellectually, but now I feel it at a primitive, visceral level.

Cindy, my original angel is continuing to be her wonderful self and keeps in touch every day. Lynne, Davida, Margot, Denise, Elaine, Celia and Evelyn, also special friends, are doing the same. The twelve friends from our play-reading group, which has been going for close on forty years, are phoning and emailing regularly, as are a bunch of other friends and Martin's brother. The reality, though, is that we are in the wrong demographic – all of our friends are working and leading exceptionally busy and demanding lives – our contact, loving as it is, is usually by necessity over the phone or internet. I yearn for physical presence: the village-closeness of friends within walking distance, able to be physically there and enfolding me.

This longing for a physical presence is tangible. Electronic communication, heartfelt as it is, carries a level of abstraction, of remoteness. I have never experienced such hunger for a friend's physical presence before, even though I have missed friends when they have been away or when I have been out of contact. The wish feels almost primitive, rooted in some non-verbal, even preverbal need. I am not surprised when, years later, I come across a piece of research measuring the levels of the stress hormone cortisol in children over a four-day period. Even when children reported stressful events, if they had a friend with them their cortisol levels were significantly lower than those in children experiencing similar events without the presence of a friend. The researcher, William Bukowski, writes, 'Our bodies recognise that they don't have to respond so much to danger if someone is there to help'.

And so I yearn to experience this present danger within the context of the gift ideal families and unencumbered friends can give – their presence. Be it for thirty minutes, an hour, an afternoon, in a way that allows you to talk, to explore and to just be. Someone for whom you can be the priority for that particular moment, who is able to provide the cushion of their simple physical presence.

My darling Amantha is here, of course, but I try to protect her, in the same way I am protecting Martin. I tell her the positive possibilities about outcomes, not the other side of the story, the one I know only too well is the more likely possibility. I don't lean on her with my fears – she is stressed enough as it is and I want to protect her.

This wish to have someone to lean on is not the need for a therapist and not even really the need to lean. It is the yen to have someone who is simply able to be there with you, although there is little that is simple about that. It is hard to stay empathically with someone who may be inhabiting a fear-filled darkness. We all want to shy away from grief, pretend it will go away or shoo it on its way with cries of 'It will be all right. It will be fine'. If we stay too long in its presence, it may pick up our identifying details, steal the keys to our house and getaway car – it is the most skilful of uninvited guests – and the places we thought so safe will be invaded too. It takes courage to stay still while it eyes us and whispers, 'You too. You too' – but staying still, staying with it, is what is needed, for however short a time.

I am at the beginning of my story but I am reminded of the ending of another story, a far older story, one of the first ever to be written down, which has reached us in shards of poetry that are 4,000 years old. It is the story of Inanna, the Sumerian Goddess of the Morning Star and Light – Inanna, the Queen of Heaven and Earth, who has decided to journey to the Underworld ruled by her sister Ereshkigal, Goddess of Darkness, Death and the World No More. No one, not even Inanna, can travel to Ereshkigal's kingdom without paying a price, and Inanna does. By the end of her journey downwards, she has been reduced by Ereshkigal to a green rotting corpse hanging on a hook.

Ereshkigal, who lives in the darkness and whose rage has turned her lips black and her face yellow, is a vastness of hate and fury when the two beings who have been assigned to rescue Inanna arrive. They have been made by Enki, God of Wisdom and Water, and they are tiny, smaller than flies, but he has told them what to do.

46

'Go to Ereshkigal', he has ordered. 'You will find her moaning with pain, with the cries of a woman about to give birth. Cry out with her. Echo her lamentations. Hear her pain'.

And they do. When they arrive, Ereshkigal is in agony: 'Oh! Oh, my inside!' she cries. 'Oh! Oh, my outside!'

And the two tiny creatures echo her: 'Oh! Oh, your inside! Oh! Oh, your outside!'

Ereshkigal, who is so feared that her own people dare not look at her and only rarely speak of her, is shocked out of her pains. These minute, inconsequential creatures have heard her suffering. Never before has this happened. She is filled with grateful amazement. So touched is she that her pain has been witnessed, she will give them anything. Even Inanna.

It is moving to have this voice from the deep past, from the time when stories were first written down thousands of years before our modern lives, remind us so clearly of what is needed in the presence of pain.

12 June 2009

It is now Martin's third day at Aberdon. I cross the threshold brightly, expecting that the physios, speechies and OTs (occupational therapists) will have got their act together and be out in force, compensating for yesterday's absence. No such luck. Amantha and I continue to fulfil our roles as speechie and physio in loco. Martin is a little impatient with us – we lack the gravitas of the real thing but we get there. Martin still cannot utter a syllable and we are communicating in whatever non-verbal ways we can muster – gestures and drawings seem to be the only language to which we have access. We are beginning to think of ourselves as the charade championship team. I feel a deep regret for never having schooled myself in the additional non-verbal languages of flags, flowers, sign or Morse.

During the day, I make numerous visits to the reception desk asking for the rehab consultant, whose name I find out is Estelle, but whose face I am clearly forbidden to see. 'She's in meetings'. 'She's not on site'. 'She's tied up'. By the end of the evening, there has still been no sighting of either *Estelle speciosa* or associated allied health professionals.

13 June 2009

With the continuing absence of allied health professionals, I have realised that further action is called for. Assertiveness has never been my forte but politeness, patience and repetition are clearly falling short of what is required to breach the Aberdon defences. I psych myself up and approach the front desk with the steam-pouring-out-of-ears expression that seems appropriate.

'I need to see Estelle'.

'She's at a meeting'.

'Well, the second she is out of that meeting, she'll be seeing me – I've been trying to see her for three days now and it's not good enough'. This last delivered with a snarl that I don't have to pretend to feel.

Within thirty minutes, the patter of consultant's feet is heard in the corridor. Estelle is coming towards me, smiling, with her hand warmly outstretched.

'Hi, I'm Estelle', she says.

'Hi, I'm Dr Brett', I reply.

Miraculous change of attitude. Estelle is all helpfulness and within an hour Martin has magically been visited by speechies, physios and OTs.

Even though they are now making an appearance, the quality and quantity of allied health professionals that Aberdon offers leave much to be desired. South-Central Rehab, with its intensive rehabilitation program, is where he needs to be.

The back-and-forth phone calls between me and South-Central are continuing, with both increasing frequency and decreasing effectiveness. I am desperate to get Martin into South-Central with its first-class therapies. We are in its catchment. The only problem is that we have been caught by Aberdon first.

I speak endlessly to managers, receptionists, supervisors, intake organisers. Nothing yields results. We tick all the boxes that would normally put us high on the waiting list but the fact that Martin already has a bed, albeit an hour's drive away, has labelled us non-urgent.

Someone tells me that if I have a personal contact at South-Central, they can help to see that Martin's case is at least reviewed for possible transfer. I ask around, but no one it seems has a personal contact at South-Central. I decide to make my next phone call that personal contact.

Up till now I have been calm and rational on the phone. This time, I decide, I will cry. I will have to turn on my inner thespian, an action that feels acutely uncomfortable for me. I love acting when reading a play or on stage, but it feels totally wrong in real life. On my next phone call to South-Central I am transferred to the assistant who handles intakes. I explain my predicament – Martin is in the catchment area of South-Central; I have a bad back and the travelling is painful for me; I don't know what to do – and at this point I let my voice waver and a sob enter it. The woman responds immediately and empathically to this. She will look again at the listings for beds, she says, and will do everything she can to get Martin in there. I thank her profusely, my voice quavering. I hang up feeling extraordinarily guilty for those manipulating sobs. I console myself with the thought that they are not really lies but rather time displacements – I do in fact sob in the late evenings, just by myself and not on the phone.

Martin by now is rallying around and starting to take his rehab seriously, the bulk of which, however, is still being conducted by the pseudo-speech therapist in the person of me and the pseudo-physio in the person of Amantha. He is still unable to speak or write, and we are focusing on the tasks of pointing to printed words, phrases and pictures.

Aberdon has a room equipped with a computer and internet access, and we take Martin on a visit, hoping that the computer, with its visuals and language that are second nature to him, will stir memories. Martin smiles when he sees the computer, sits down in front of it, reaches his good hand towards the keyboard and then suddenly freezes – he does not know what to do. He does not know even the first simple thing to do.

In the late evenings at home, I am experiencing a similar state. What is flooring me is the mass of practical financial issues I have persistently failed to learn about over the years. Although our earning power has been fairly similar and I have always worked except for a privileged time when Amantha was a toddler, daily financial management has been Martin's arena. Over the last few years, I have thought many times that I needed to learn about the paperwork, the bill-filing, the tax-return forms and the other assorted financial paperwork. I have thought it. And then I have thought, 'I'll learn about it tomorrow'. It is part laziness, part fatigue, part habit and partly the fact that Martin does it so supremely well and is happy to claim it as his sphere.

I am horrified by how little I know. I am a preschooler attempting a PhD. Even internet banking is a mystery to me and, with my Luddite tendencies, I have never used an ATM. I feel humiliatingly feeble, and my stupidity and slackness in this area feel shameful. This is all heightened by the fact that in order to access ATMs, internet banking and the like, we need a pin number or password. I don't know the password and pin. Martin knows the password and pin. But Martin cannot speak or write. And all the bills are starting to come in, arriving like the migrating birds of another hemisphere, as June gets underway. I don't have the money at hand. I cannot access the online banking system without a password and I cannot even get to the bank in person as I am spending from dawn till dusk with Martin at Aberdon. Luckily, Amantha is able to lend me the money to cover the bills. It is a sobering and frightening experience. I feel inept, incompetent and embarrassingly stupid.

Bill-paying is further inhibited by the fact that the Visa card I use for online transactions was stolen just a few days before Martin's stroke. The bank was supposed to issue a replacement pronto, but pronto has clearly lost something of its definition in the bank's dictionary and the new card has still not made an appearance.

It is now a week since Martin's stroke, although the attempt to frame this experience in units of time seems akin to the task of describing a banana using only the characteristics of an elephant. Time and Martin's illness seem totally disconnected. Days have melted and stretched in a way that has nothing to do with clocks. Their external shape is always the same – the early morning drive into Frankston, the late evening drive back – but the time in between seems beyond measurement, as if it existed in a separate universe. The familiar internal accounting of hours that we note without thinking in normal daily life has vanished. Time is a different animal in illness, at times stretched beyond the view of horizons, at others shrinking to micro-size.

With the new body clock that an immersion in terror brings, I am finding myself awake at times when everyone else is asleep. This, the solitary dead-of-night territory of insomniacs, is when I have a particular longing to experience the aliveness of talking to another human being. In this, the computer, once my bête noire, is now my saviour. Through it I can communicate and connect, even when everyone I know is asleep. In one way this sense of connecting is illusory – no one is reading this as I write it – but in another, it is absolutely real. I know that in a few hours someone will indeed be reading my words, will be 'hearing' my voice. My words are not just silent messages to myself. Come morning, they will reach another's ears.

Writing these group updates to friends has become an essential part of my nightly routine. I never miss an update, and although I know they are important to me, I have no idea how deep their comfort is until now, when quite suddenly, at four in the dark hours of very early morning, as I am typing away, the computer suddenly and without warning freezes.

I run through my repertoire of computer solutions. Solutions, plural, is overstating it – my repertoire consists of rebooting. And rebooting some more. And still nothing happens. The screen remains frozen. I cannot move the cursor. I cannot read incoming mail. I cannot send off outgoing mail. If Martin were here he would be able to fix it in minutes. But Martin is miles away, unreachable and in his own way as frozen as the computer.

I tap at the keys more forcefully but the screen remains inert. It is a wall, its electronic blankness cutting me off completely and utterly from that automatic, entitled interface I have come to assume between my brain and the distant transmission of words. Communication has been severed. I am without a voice.

And suddenly I am cracked through with disconnection. Not just the disconnection of the computer. The computer is also the hospital, the stroke, the precariousness of the future – everything from the last week that is now hitting me with the thwack of a wrecking ball. The civilised part of my mind is blanked out – the reasoning part, the one that tells me what I have to do and how I have to do it, the one that thinks, researches, plans and works out ways to cope, blinks out like a light and I start to howl. It is a sound I have never made before in my life. It is not crying, not weeping, not sobbing, not keening, not wailing or any one of the dozens of words used to describe the sounds of sorrow. It is howling, a sound defined by the dictionary as 'a long, doleful cry uttered by an animal such as a dog or wolf'. And that is what I am. The animal separated from its pack, the child lost in the supermarket – enveloped by the first fear we have when we come into the world unshelled and vulnerable – the unbearable, unutterable fear of the abandoned, the lost, the never-to-be-found.

After a while the howling stops. I am exhausted. I have an overpowering need, a compulsion really, to talk to someone – but it is only 4.00 am. I cannot wake a friend at this hour. I go through a list of friends, computing who is an early riser, who gets up early for work and what is the earliest time I can decently ring them.

And then, Davida! Davida is a dear and special friend and Davida is in America. I calculate California time and it is daylight there. I dial. My fingers are shaky – I hit the wrong buttons and have to keep correcting myself. But when I finally get the right combination of numbers, the phone rings into answering machine mode – she is not home.

I work out that the nearest decent time I can ring anyone is 8.00 am, four hours away. The clock crawls and I pace like a demented woman, overcome by this desperation, this necessity, to speak with someone, to connect with someone, with another human being who knows me and cares about me. Finally, it is a quarter to eight and I can ring Elaine. Within seconds I am myself again. Normal again. Distressed but normal. It is the only time I have this unnerving experience, but I know now that it is there. Certainly for me. Maybe for everyone. The infinity of black water under the ice.

14 June 2009

In the normalising light of day, although the memory of what was laid bare is still with me, the computer problem takes on the shape of what it is – a computer problem. Vexing, deeply frustrating but not the last lifeboat off the *Titanic*. Martin understands when I tell him that the computer has frozen and that I cannot restart it, but he shrugs his shoulders helplessly.

In his normal life Martin is a highly talented computer analyst, but in this life, he is impotent. Amantha and I play twenty questions with him about what cyber-intervention might be needed, but nothing emerges. Martin is now able to make a slightly wider variety of vocal sounds but still cannot enunciate even the most simple of words. He signals for a piece of paper and, with his left hand, laboriously manages to scrawl a few letters – the first few of which resemble 'mond'.

'Monday?' we ask eagerly and he nods vigorously.

'Should we do something on Monday?'

His head shakes no.

'Is something happening on Monday?'

He nods yes.

'Will someone be in an office on Monday we should contact?'

Headshake, no.

'Will something happen to the computer on Monday?'

An excited nod, yes – we have finally got it.

'Do we have to do anything on Monday?'

Headshake, no.

Amantha and I are mystified about what will happen, seemingly automatically, to the computer on Monday, but Martin seems certain that the turning of the calendar date will do the trick.

I spend that evening unsuccessfully applying various suggested computer remedies. Nothing works. My computer remains stubbornly retired from the cyber rat-race.

Apart from the difficulty this causes me in researching, I feel a ripping sense of loss in being unable to read friends' emails written in response to my daily updates. And an even deeper sense of displacement in being unable to write and send off the group updates.

I have always thought I was relatively independent of the cyber-world. I am not on Facebook. I don't use Twitter. I check my email sparingly. I have occasionally read stories of people who are going cold turkey in an effort to see what life is like without all their constant cyber-stimulation and I have felt superior. No longer. I am discovering I am as dependent as they are. My range of dependency is narrower but the need is as intense. I have to communicate. And currently email is the only way I can communicate at any length with friends who are on the move through busy days.

And so, despite the fact that I am in the world, albeit it the micro-world of Aberdon, I feel torn away from it – a shipwreck survivor whose last means of communicating with the shore has disappeared. The intensity of this feeling is striking – in reality I still have the phone, the car and I can still write for myself in the old-fashioned pen-and-pencil way. But with my days and evenings spent corralled in the telecommunications black hole of Aberdon and the ultra-packed busyness of modern life, managing contact with friends is far harder than I imagined it would be. And more and more I am realising that I am writing the updates not just to put down my thoughts, but to be read. And by that I must mean to be heard, to have my human presence and experience understood and listened to by another, not just myself, that ancient, hardwired human need for connection.

Amantha organises a method for me to send and receive via her computer. It is an extraordinary relief to be able to communicate again, to be connected in a way that feels much deeper than I could ever previously have imagined.

From what my limited wits can gather, in order to activate Martin's computer (the big and controlling brother of my smaller unit), which has gone on strike in a chicken-and-egg manoeuvre with its sibling, we need Martin's password. And here, of course, I run into the familiar problem. Only Martin knows Martin's password and Martin cannot communicate. I have explained all this endlessly to the telcos but they are adamant – the only way to activate the computer is through Martin's password. I look through Martin's filing cabinet as best I can, but cannot find any reference to a password and quite likely couldn't recognise it even if I saw it. Walter, a computer-savvy friend, offers to come over and see if he can inveigle the computer into starting up again and I am deeply appreciative.

Walter presses various buttons, rings telcos and has arcane conversations with the techs on the other end, but the result is the same. Nada, nothing, zilch. The helplessness is profound. I have allowed myself to become utterly dependent on something of which I have not even the slightest understanding. I have traded understanding for convenience and speed and now I am hostage to it.

No one has any idea what significance Monday has for computer health, but it seems to be all we have to hold onto. I make regular attempts to get my computer to unfreeze – I press keys, speak to it, yell at it, threaten and plead. It remains unflickering and inert. It is not like talking to a brick wall – brick walls have nothing going on inside them; even on their best days they are unlikely to respond. It is more like talking to a person in a drunken coma – they are non-responsive but you cannot help feeling that it is possible to rouse them if you just do this, and then this, and this. The poker-machine fallacy – where the next press you make might just be the right one. And so I am unable to restrain myself from going up the stairs to try 'just one more time' again and again and again.

Update, 15 June 2009

I am writing this via Amantha's computer, mine having decided to take an unscheduled break from the work-force. Not unlike the Aberdon staff, it is present in body but not in spirit.

Martin's nurse yesterday was a delightful character who is convinced we are all just exceptionally tall two-year-olds and addresses us accordingly. She puts on her best 'storytelling' voice and does a remarkable imitation of Mrs Marsh in that ancient but memorable commercial where she demonstrates to the children that yes, chalk is exactly like the enamel of our teeth and when you dip it into ink (and we all like our occasional tipple of ink) it turns dark.

This nurse also has a belief in paranormal communication. At 6.00 am yesterday morning, she helped Martin print out on a piece of paper, 'Bring soap'. The idea was to convey this message telepathically so that the charade team would automatically add it to their list before they set out from home in the morning. When we arrived without soap and requested some, she looked astonished at a) the fact that we did not receive the message, and b) the possibility that the hospital might have to supply this essential product.

A few hours later I noticed that Martin had an open sore on his hand. I pointed it out to nurse number two. 'Yes', she said, with the vague interest of an artist commenting on a rather derivative painting, 'I'd been noticing that'. I offered the thought that a bandaid might be helpful. 'Oh, we don't do bandaids', she replied airily.

An old Marx Brothers anecdote concerns a buffet party given by Harpo. Guests partaking of the feast were dismayed to find an absence of serviettes. Hearing the grumbles, Oscar Levant stood to make an announcement: 'Due to the high cost of living, there are no napkins, but from time to time a woolly dog will pass amongst you'.

Clearly Aberdon has subscribed to the same principle.

Last night I put out a saucer of milk and bread and was eagerly anticipating the arrival of the Monday Computer Fairy. With the way I have been sleeping, I expected to be up to hear the rustle of her wings and the delicate tapping of her wand on the keyboard as our computer magically reformed itself.

In the early hours of this morning, I made a quiet foray upstairs, hoping to surprise the Computer Fairy in the act. Alas... The first clue that all was not well was the fact that the saucer of bread and milk I had carefully laid out for the Fairy (books on Celtic folklore had been intensively consulted to ascertain the most appropriate offering) was untouched. My heart sank, but I pressed on, hoping that perhaps it was simply that the Fairy was on a diet. Sad to say, however, the fairy hadn't come. An explanation was forthcoming for her absence, however (thank you Denise) – Denise informed me (too late, unfortunately) that the problem was I had neglected to sprinkle hundreds and thousands onto the bread. In the end we had to give up and buy the Telstra Fairy instead, who comes complete with her own new modem in a few days.

Martin is continuing to improve slowly – he is walking, albeit a touch unsteadily, and the number of sounds he can make is increasing, although he still cannot speak. He can understand everything, he just cannot express himself either through speech or writing. He has been taking an alert interest in the computer problem and appears to be sure that he knows the answer but just cannot communicate it. It is strange to see the disconnect between the thoughts that are obviously going on in his head and his ability to express them.

16 June 2009

When I make my regular call to Aberdon before setting out this morning, I receive the exhilarating news that Martin is being transferred to South-Central Rehabilitation Hospital today. The ambulance will take him to South-Central and I will meet him there. I am as excited as a winner on a TV quiz show. South-Central is where he will have what he needs by way of expert speech and physiotherapy. South-Central is where the work will begin.

The South-Central campus is huge. I used to work at an adjoining clinic decades ago and have memories of getting lost in the big hospital's rabbit warrens on my occasional excursions there. It is an old hospital. Old in the non-quaint way. Peeling walls, ancient five-bed wards that have stepped straight out of the 1930s, and an overall sense of dilapidation. I find my way to Martin's section of the hospital and the 'common room', where I have been told to meet him.

I am directed to a small room with some chairs, a table and a scattering of very elderly magazines. A handful of occupants, equally elderly, are sitting around. And there is Martin.

He is in a chair, huddled into himself, looking confused and upset. As I hug him I work out that he had arrived earlier than I had been told, been seated in this chair and then just left alone, a situation that might be fine for many patients, but not for one who has no means of communicating and for whom walking is still tricky and dangerous. He had been wanting to go to the toilet but had no way of letting anyone know.

Blood boiling, I find a nurse who takes Martin off to the toilets. I also enquire about where the women's version is and am told just to use the communal one. One look inside persuades me I can keep my bladder under control for a while yet.

A few hours pass before Martin is allotted a bed. As we walk slowly in the direction indicated, I keep my fingers crossed that it is not one of the dingy, cramped five-bed wards I glimpsed on the way in. Alas, Martin is indeed in the Hieronymus Bosch ward. As I look around, it is clear the hospital is missing out on lucrative fundraising possibilities by not hiring itself out to aspiring horror filmmakers.

Martin's bed is in the middle of a ward inhabited by brain-damaged elderly men. His diagonally opposite neighbour, whose name appears to be Trevor, keeps getting up, throwing off his clothes and wandering naked around the ward, showering all with urine as he goes. This continues with relentless regularity throughout the day. As does my haring off to fetch a nurse, since Trevor is not supposed to be walking.

17 June 2009

For the first time Martin's mood is flat – he cannot sleep due to the noisy conditions (four varieties of all-night snorers) and Trevor, whose wanderings don't stop with the going down of the sun. Trevor is so disruptive during the night that no one in the ward gets any sleep. In a place where sick people have come to be healed, the deprivation of sleep, so necessary for the repair of the body and mind, is shocking. Of course, South-Central is not alone in this flaw – it is echoed in hospitals everywhere.

The ward is dark, old and correspondingly grubby. I have scouted my way along the corridor and discovered that a few doors down is a three-bed ward that looks light-filled and comparatively airy. I am determined to get Martin into it.

To this end, I arrive at the nurses' station with a box of chocolates along with the plea for a bed transfer. Their replies are vague and ambiguous – enough to encourage more chocolates but not enough for contractual certainty. And of course no time frame is given or even implied. It is a seller's market. I determine to keep bringing chocolates and pleas until it happens.

I am also waiting for the rehab consultant's visit, both to hear his assessment of Martin's condition and to put in a bed request. I was told he did rounds at 8.30 am, so I arrive there at 8.00 am to be certain. Of course there has been no sign of him, and it seems now he will not come at all today. Martin's program hasn't started yet, so I have brought in some pages of the elementary word exercises I was using at Aberdon. In between doing these and chatting to Martin, I watch the unfolding of the hospital day.

The nurses are clearly wildly overworked. They are dealing with deeply incapacitated patients and are understaffed as well. Some of the men in Martin's ward take themselves off to their various rehab therapists during the day, but Trevor remains in situ and the regular Trevor round-up continues. Every fifteen minutes without fail he sheds his clothes, sometimes onto Martin's bed, and lurches around the ward like a misshapen and malfunctioning fountain, the South-Central version of Belgium's *Manneken Pis*.

My initial reaction of horrified pity has now deteriorated to a much less saintly one of intense frustration as I continue to see the disturbing impact he has on his ward-mates. And in particular on Martin who, for some unknown reason, has now had his bed shifted so that he is right next to Trevor. This results in encounters of the horror-movie kind for unsuspecting visitors.

This afternoon, while Walter is visiting, Trevor's naked arm, with clawed, curled skeletal fingers, suddenly shoots out of the curtain almost into Martin's face with an impact that Hitchcock could only envy. Walter, who is a grown man and sound of mind, nearly screams.

18 June 2009

Today I suddenly notice a distinct absence of Trevor. On investigation, which involves cautiously peering through a large chink in his curtain, I realise it is because he has a nurse sitting with him full-time on the evening shift in an understaffed ward. My increasingly violent and politically incorrect fantasies regarding what to do about Trevor do not include taking up the services of a whole nurse who is so badly needed by the rest of the wards.

This Trevor-free condition, however, will last only through tonight. By tomorrow, both Trevor and my fetch-the-nurse aerobic activities will be back at full throttle.

Martin will also be getting the outlines of his therapy program tomorrow. It will be so heartening to have the sense of something happening. He still cannot speak at all and his mood has been bleak – not surprising, given his current surroundings. Martin likes the comforts of home. He doesn't like camping. He doesn't even particularly like travelling and the inconveniences of hotel rooms. It is nightmarish for him to have landed in the blighted environment of this five-bed ward with its barely adequate bathroom facilities, no privacy, no peace and with no ability even to communicate. I am with him during the day and can shield him from some of this but at night when I am not there, he is totally vulnerable.

19 June 2009

It is now Martin's third day at South-Central and above his bed hangs a timetable of physio, speech and occupational therapy sessions. It resembles a weekly university lecture timetable and each day is structured a little differently. They are planning on keeping Martin busy and for the first time since this all began, I am not needed by his side as he takes on his new work routine. It is strange to be leaving Martin alone for long periods of time. I feel oddly like the mother of a preschooler dropping her child off to the institutional care of strangers for the first time. And during the two-hour breaks that are part of each day, I arrive, complete with food treats, and read the speech therapist's notes to find out what happened 'in class' today.

I have also now met Charles, the rehabilitation consultant. He arrived with his team trailing him at 8.30 am this morning. Right time, wrong day, according to yesterday's nurse informant. He is approachable, easy to talk to and looks as if he is barely old enough to graduate from high school, let alone obtain a specialist medical degree. He will be the ultimate authority on all things Martin-related at South-Central.

The team have had a meeting to discuss their initial assessments of Martin, and Charles gives me the lowdown. Obviously, Martin's stroke has left him severely disabled and progress will require intensive work. The duration of the average stay at South-Central is variable, and at Aberdon they had told us to expect four weeks. The team, however, thinks six weeks will be a better option for Martin and, as Charles relays this news, I can see Martin's face fall. I can understand his expression. Six hours in these surroundings is taxing, six weeks seems unimaginable.

Charles is guarded in his prognosis. The most he will say is that they hope Martin will recover some speech, although they don't expect he will get even remotely close to his past fluency. His right arm is still paralysed from the shoulder down and his right leg is still weak, although he can walk slowly, and rather unsteadily, and needs someone beside him. Physio will be working on those issues and again, the prognosis for that is unknown.

As soon as the team has departed, I bring out my usual speech about brain plasticity and an excellent recovery. Although I infuse my voice with confidence and authority, in fact, from everything I know, the odds of this happening are not good. I have two friends who are speech pathologists and another who is a neuropsychologist.

When we talk, we conclude that although it is possible, the odds of Martin making an excellent recovery are vastly outranked by the probability that he will not.

I don't share this knowledge with either Martin or Amantha. Martin has such taxing work ahead of him that to approach it without hope is to doom it before it even starts. And Amantha has a demanding business to run as well as the shock of her father's illness to deal with – it is enough that this frightening knowledge is carried by only one of us.

The state of Martin's ward-mates underlines this sense of pessimism. They have all suffered strokes and many of them have been at South-Central for weeks without making noticeable progress. They are starting to resolve themselves into separate personalities rather than a conglomeration of elderly disabled men.

Diagonally across from Martin on the left is an English gentleman who gallantly flirts with the nurses, but in fact has very little comprehension of what is going on. I am reminded of Alice, desperately trying to apply her old rules of how to behave in society to the crazy, upside-down world she has fallen into.

The bed across to Martin's right contains a man who is in for his third stroke. I made his acquaintance yesterday evening when he suddenly began to sob loudly. I went over to talk to him and see if I could do anything and his story emerged. His wife died three years ago and he lives alone. He has two daughters – the older one is a cold-hearted, selfish creature, the younger one a sweetheart, and the two girls will not talk to each other. He is desperate to go on day leave so he can buy himself a personal computer to use while in hospital. Because of his health, he is only allowed to leave the hospital with a chaperone. His younger daughter is willing to take him but cannot get away from work. His older daughter doesn't work but is unwilling to take him to the shop. As we talk, his sobs die down and he begins telling me more about himself.

He is Costas, a builder from Greece, who was once an aspiring novelist. He seems an intelligent, capable man who is enormously frustrated by the dependence this stroke has thrust upon him. For him, the stroke has hit his motor abilities. He can walk, but is unsteady and not allowed to drive, hence his dependence on his daughters. No friends ever visit and he is obviously lonely. I make a point of going over to chat to him regularly.

The other beds are inhabited by men who, although less active than Trevor, seem to be functioning at around the same level as him. One lucky man has landed the best bed in the ward – the one on the end by the window. It is almost in its own alcove, with only one, instead of two, neighbouring beds. He spends most of the time with his curtain drawn, thus giving himself the illusion of a private room along with the addition of sunshine from the window.

For much of his time in both Frankston and Aberdon hospitals, Martin was remarkably calm. Since coming to South-Central, however, his mood has deteriorated to morose and surly. When he has visitors, he smiles, but when I walk into the room, there is not even a micro-lift of his mouth. I can understand it absolutely. South-Central is hell and so is his situation. At times like this, those closest usually become the cat kicked in frustration while others get smiles and politeness. But his grumpiness is showing itself in his speech sessions. He is impatient, uninterested and not working well.

Feeling like a nasty Big Brother, I decide I have to give him a pep talk. It is made even more hypocritical by the fact that I know, were I in his position, I would be howling, screaming and sobbing without pause. But South-Central is his big chance to work at recovery. He cannot blow it with a 'can't be bothered' attitude. He has to be bothered.

I have a little internal discussion with myself about timing. Obviously, Martin is entitled to blowing-off-steam days and equally entitled to feel miserable, angry and self-pitying – who wouldn't in his situation? But how long is too long? Am I expecting too much of him? Should I just wait it out? But these early days in South-Central will set patterns for his relationships with his therapists and for his own sense of self. His surroundings are guaranteed to promote depression and irritability but if he can be nudged or even jolted back to a sense of working determinedly and optimistically, he will be buoyed and energised by his achievements.

And so I decide that three days of this is enough. He listens sullenly to what I have to say and I finish by giving him a hug as he gets picked up for his speech session. I walk back to his room feeling like an utter heel.

But it works. Martin is escorted back from his speech session all smiles. The speech pathologist tells me that for the first time he had a terrific session and really worked hard. She is enthusiastic, he is pleased and excited. I nearly sink to my knees with relief.

And from that point on, Martin's attitude to his work never flags. I am overwhelmed with admiration at the positive and persistent way he attacks his work, no matter how frustrating, no matter how small the gains.

He has now, for the first time, started to be able to shape certain sounds. I sit in on one of his speech sessions. Whereas we make these sounds without thinking, Martin has to learn the most basic mechanics of how to create them. He has to learn what shape to curve his lips into, where to place his tongue, which of the muscles in his mouth to move and in what sequence and how to coordinate all of these movements with his breath in order to make just one specific sound. As almost all words consist of multiple sounds, even one-syllable words such as 'yes', the mechanics of speaking even one word, let alone a sentence, require sustained concentration and intense learning. His brain has simply lost the connections that tell it how to do this automatically. While I watch throughout the hour-long session, he haltingly manages to pronounce two different sounds – 'b' and 'd'.

With his newly learned skills, Martin can now slowly and painfully pronounce a handful of simple words. It is both torturous to watch and at the same time unutterably exciting.

Martin's brain has also forgotten how to transform the words in his head into the written symbols on paper that represent them. But he is also starting to make progress in this area – he is now beginning to be able to transcribe a few words onto paper. He writes with his left hand, of course, as his right hand is still paralysed, but he can now write a word or two. In someone without spoken language, the ability to write even one word can be a godsend in helping to communicate.

Update, 19 June 2009

Martin stunned his speech therapist today with a sterling performance and stunned author of update too when she rang at night and requested nurse to put her through to Martin so she could tell him she had reminded the nurse to give him his sleeping tablets – Martin's voice was strong and author could make out a couple of words quite clearly, including 'hello' – a dramatic improvement over yesterday.

The reason I was reminding the nurse about sleeping tablets was that they forgot last night. 'Does he really need sleeping tablets?' the nurse asked me. 'His bed is next door to Trevor's', I said. 'Understood', she replied. Nurses have responded to the Trevor problem by doping him to the gills. I only had to play the 'Catch the Trevor, Tell the Nurses' game a couple of times, when he heroically overcame the effects of drugs that could stop a racehorse in its tracks and staggered to his feet in pre-lurch.

I am sick with a viral bug, with symptoms that include a strange rash. Am so spacey that I hadn't even noticed rash until I went to GP, who pointed out that I actually had a rash over my entire body. And in fact I now look more like fairy bread than fairy bread.

Martin's CT scan results, which I finally managed to chase up, showed there may or may not be a vascular malformation in Martin's brain and he may or may not need neurosurgery and it may or may not be operable. CT scans have been sent to the Prince Edward neurosurgeons, who will look at them on Monday. I am hoping this might-be-there-might-not-be phenomenon will prove a phantom – they are looking hard for something and it may be that they are seeing things where they are not to be seen. Fingers crossed, anyway.

After ferrying myself to the doctor for my bug, I then had to ferry poor Amantha, who is also sick and was running a temp. We both have coughs and so as well as being the charade championship team we have plans for another skill set – if we meet anyone who displeases us, at a given signal we will coordinate-cough all over them.

And in an amazing development, Walter made another attempt to resuscitate my computer and this time it responded. My computer is working again!

20 June 2009

It is hard to believe that it is two weeks since this all began. It is actually still hard to believe that it all began.

Martin has had a terrific two days in terms of his speech progress – he is definitely improving at a faster rate. His smile is back to its usual brilliant self and he has a fantastic attitude – the speech therapist underlined 'really' in the 'really good' in her report. Martin's walking is much better and his writing is improving. When I rang him last night I could make out some clear words in a way I hadn't been able to before.

I have also discovered a wonderful budgie aviary close to Martin's ward and walked him over there this morning – huge aviary and dozens of gorgeously coloured birds having a great and extremely social time. Mesmerising and beautiful to watch. So wonderful to have in the midst of the very grungy old South-Central wards.

Trevor is continuing to be stuffed to the gills with tranquillisers – in today's somewhat frozen posture, he rather resembles an old-time dime-store wooden Indian and could perhaps make a decorative addition to any establishment requiring a focal interior-decorating statement.

22 June 2009

Denise has joined me for an evening visit to Martin. He is cheerful at the sight of visitors and Denise chats to him about some of the new dances she is teaching. We have just returned to the house when the phone rings. I pick it up, expecting it to be a friend enquiring about Martin. Instead, what I hear is an anguished, inhuman scream in which no words can be distinguished.

It takes shocked seconds before I realise this terrifying sound must be Martin.

'Martin', I say, racing through all the horrific possibilities of what could have gone wrong.

Again, no words, only a primeval scream of distress.

'Are you in pain? What's wrong?' My frantic questions are an automatic reflex – with Martin unable to speak, I have no possibility of them being answered.

The same anguished scream again. Sounding worse, if anything.

'I'm coming', I say. 'It's okay, I'm coming'.

Denise and I jump into the car and together we make our way through the pitch-darkness of the hospital's back entrance car park – stumbling as we try to run without the benefit of sight and burning with the anxiety of what those screams might signify.

In the ward I find Martin almost jumping out of his skin with distress. He is tugging at his pyjamas and making the same wordless grunts and shrieks I heard on the phone. After a frenzy of frantic gestures and pantomimes, I finally realise that what has upset him is his wish for fresh pyjamas.

'I'll be right back with some', I say, and Denise and I race crazily back to the car.

In the house, I grab as many pyjamas as I can find. Martin calms when I present them and help him get into a pair. I am just relaxing into feeling the crisis has been managed when his face crumples again. He shows me one foot with a sock on and one foot without.

I rummage in his bag and manage to find another sock, not the pair to the one he has on. But Martin shakes his head violently. No, he wants the socks to be properly paired.

'Just for tonight?' I plead, but he refuses. For whatever reason, this is paramount to him.

I am stuck, trying to think of a solution that doesn't involve yet another trip back home and to the hospital.

Suddenly I realise that what he wants is two socks of the same colour. I slip off my shoes, take off my own socks and present them to him.

He nods happily and I help him put them on. He then sinks back, utterly exhausted.

It is only long afterwards that I realise that somehow, in the midst of this foggy, wordless distress, Martin has remembered not only how to use the phone but the correct eight digits of our phone number.

23 June 2009

The bed the nurse has promised me for Martin is due to be vacated this morning – it is the coveted end bed by the window. I am beside myself with excitement and determined to get into the ward at the crack of dawn to supervise Martin's transfer to the 'good' bed.

With immaculate timing, however, the house phone doesn't stop ringing from the moment I get up. As a result, I get into the hospital an hour later than intended. Almost at a run, I approach the ward, so excited at the thought that Martin is at last going to have a modicum of privacy and space that I am practically effervescing. And then, just inside the door, I come to a dead stop. The window bed has indeed been transferred. To Costas.

I nearly cry. I have worked so hard and so long to get Martin a better bed and now it is gone. I head down to the nurses station and with some persuasion at least manage to get Martin allocated to Costas's old bed – no longer next door to Trevor.

As I talk to the nurses, the story emerges. Costas had heard me telling Martin that the best bed in the ward was being vacated on Monday and that the charge nurse had promised it to Martin. Costas then got vocal this morning as soon as he saw it vacated (Martin, of course, cannot get vocal) and insisted on being moved to that bed. The charge nurse told me she was at morning tea when this happened and didn't find out until he was already in it. Costas already had the second best bed in the ward (while Martin had the worst), but he obviously intended to grab the best bed for himself regardless of who it had been promised to. So, no more sympathy for Costas. It seems particularly underhanded given how much I have gone out of my way to be good to him.

Earlier this morning while it was still dark, I had woken sweating from a stressful dream. I had been chasing and trying to kill a shiny, hard-shelled beetle. Frantically, I kept trying to step on it but it always escaped. Suddenly I knew stepping on it wouldn't work because a voice kept saying urgently, 'The sole won't do it. The sole won't do it'. The beetle got away while I panted helplessly and finally woke.

And at eleven o'clock this morning, I discover that something else has got away from me. My mobile phone. It is physically present but otherwise absent. Repeatedly I dial from every spot in the house and surroundings. Every attempt is met with the ping of the 'call failed' message. It is utterly and unreasoningly maddening. I am so used to my brain's will flowing seamlessly through my fingertips and into the phone that the ping of the failed message feels like a personal insult. An electronic finger salute that says, 'You are helpless. You have no control'. I try again and again, hoping to find that one small inch of territory that allows the message to be completed. As I fail repeatedly, I begin to realise that in some small way this is the miniaturised echo of Martin's experience of his brain impotently signalling his paralysed right arm.

The failure of my phone also means that in the two weeks since Martin's stroke, every technological device that I depend on for my connection to the world has failed – my missing Visa card, my computer and now my phone. Every hour of my day is spent either with Martin or with patients in that cut-off, isolated universe into which carers of very ill people are thrown. And now I have been shut off from electronic communication with the world as well. The failure of this phone feels insanely like the last portal to the world slamming shut, as if the universe is insisting that the world of the ill remain separate – that there is no easy passage between it and the land of the well.

I spend a good deal of today in the oxymoronic world of 'customer service' via the usual outposts in distant cities. First they insist that the fault is not theirs – that the problem must be in my handset, not the sim card. I take the phone down to a mobile phone shop and wait the usual hour before being served. The assistant is a young man who speaks in a tech language that may as well be the fabled Double Dutch as he effortlessly takes apart my phone, connects it to various devices and finally assures me that the fault is not in my phone, it is in the sim card and therefore the responsibility of the company from which it was bought.

As someone who has never knowingly set eyes on a sim card, let alone developed an understanding of what it is, I parrot the phrases that the young man has uttered. He nods yes and I hurry home to my landline to renew conversations with the far-flung representatives of the phone company.

To no avail. They continue to insist that it cannot possibly be their fault. My attempts to explain, first reasonably, then curtly then extremely abruptly that it is their fault, continue over several hours and a dozen more phone calls before they finally concede that yes, it is the sim card. At which point I switch to chanting, 'Either cancel my subscription or send me a new sim card'. To which they respond No. And then proceed to argue backwards that in fact although they have conceded that it is their fault, it is really not their fault.

In between all this, I am running out to be with Martin in his hours off, trying to chase down the reports from his recent brain MRI and deal with the hundred and one other tasks that need to be done urgently. Each task is essential, each task takes twice as long as I anticipate and each task has only me to do it.

As I frantically triple-, quadruple- and quintuple-task, the landline rings every twenty minutes – bland young men and women relentlessly reciting from identical scripts, agreeing that yes, it is a sim card fault, but no, it is not their fault even though they sold me the sim card and no they will not change the sim card, refund my money or solve the problem. What they want me to do is spend several more hours on the phone discussing it with them so they can say at the end of it, yes, it is the sim card and no, it is not their fault and no, they will not solve the problem.

I slam the phone down but I cannot afford to leave it off the hook – important medical calls are also coming in. I order the telco staff to stop ringing me – the matter is closed, I will buy a new phone from a different company. But the phone continues to ring again and again like a giant, demented bee. Over a dozen times more that day, I race to answer it in case it is the doctors, the hospital or the MRI reports. My voice is getting harsher, shriller, as I order them time and time again to stop ringing me.

And then, at 6.00 pm, just as I am leaving the house with Amantha to see Martin, the phone rings yet again. I race back through the house, frantic in my rush to catch it in case it is the medicos. I grab the receiver, nearly tripping as I do so, and pant my acknowledgement, only to hear the drone of the telco servants. And I lose it. For the first, and hopefully last, time in my life I start screaming and swearing over the phone. I am a fishwife, a berserker, a crazy person – the maniac on cop shows being dragged off, kicking and screaming, by the sane ones.

My phone assailant is shocked into silence. Amantha is looking at me in horror. I am just realising that the insane shrieking I can hear is coming out of me. I slam the phone down and Amantha and I look at each other in stunned silence.

I take some forced deep breaths. I am shaking with boiled-over stress and rage. I unclench my fists, make myself continue breathing and gradually, very gradually, I begin to return to myself.

The next day I organise a new phone. As Amantha shows me how to use it, she says casually, 'What company was the faulty sim card sold by?' I have no idea. I have just been dialling the number written down for me. We search the papers in Martin's file and finally find the receipt for the old phone. The company is called Soul. My dream was right – 'The sole won't do it'.

24 June 2009

I am sitting with Martin during his late morning break from therapy when Charles cruises by on his rounds. He checks that Martin is walking steadily and then startles me by saying, 'Do you want to take him home for a lunchbreak?'

Martin and I both jump out of our respective skins with shock and excitement. Home! A lunchbreak!

I bundle Martin into warm outer clothing – it is freezing winter outside – and, keeping firm hold on his good arm, help him step into the outside world for the first time since his stroke all those centuries ago.

I am so used to being inside with him, enclosed by the thick stuffiness of institutional walls, that it feels weirdly, deliriously elating to be out with him under wide skies and with real weather in our faces.

There is a fair amount of manipulating to do – taking off Martin's sling so that the seatbelt can be attached, redoing the sling to start the journey, undoing the sling on arrival, undoing the seatbelt, redoing the sling, helping him out of the car, taking care with the steps – but finally, miraculously, Martin is stepping through the door into his own home.

He wants an omelette for lunch and I am breaking the required eggs when I realise my legs feel as frail and fragile as the eggshells. I have been subsisting on three or four hours' sleep a night and am tottery with fatigue and stress. I sit down, not wanting Martin to see my unsteadiness.

Martin indicates that he wants to go upstairs to his study. I am unsure. I don't know whether he is allowed to climb stairs. His OTs have been missing in action for a few days and I have had no instructions about what he is allowed to attempt physically. In my weakened state, I am also unsure how good I will be at supporting him physically if necessary.

But Martin is adamant. He wants to go upstairs and it is clear that if I don't help him, he will do it himself. So, with Martin holding onto the banister with one hand and me holding onto Martin on the other side, we make our slow progress upwards. At his desk, Martin settles into his chair with a sigh and turns on his computer. He is home.

When I come back into the room a few minutes later, I see to my amazement that he has opened up our online bank account and is working, one slow, clumsy and often incorrect keystroke at a time, on the task of paying our bills. Less than a month ago he couldn't count to five and he still cannot speak, but he is sitting there now, step by hard-won step, paying our bills.

I take Martin back to South-Central in time for his afternoon shift of therapy, and when I return in the early evening he is still glowing, both with the thrill and the achievement of his home visit. I sit with him a while and then kiss him goodnight. As I leave the ward, a glance backwards reveals Trevor stripping off and attempting to climb into Martin's cupboard.

My days continue to be split between South-Central, whenever Martin has breaks in his schedule, and seeing patients. The odd in-between moments are spent on those routine, endless household chores that are necessities – taking the rubbish out, doing the washing, making the supermarket runs. I am busy, there is barely a moment without work to do, but I am lonely.

My professional work is solitary – I work in private practice as a psychologist. There are no work colleagues to greet or chat with. Amantha is wonderful, but my priority is protecting her. I want to keep things as normal as possible for her. When she is not working, I want her to be able to unwind and spend time with her partner in their own home. She is my daughter and, in the way of mothers of all ages, I want to take care of her. The family I long for are cousins, sisters, mothers, aunts – the family who have always known you, on whom you can lean, the ones who offer untimed, unquestioning shelter.

As a child, I had a sense of extended family. All of my mother's immediate family were murdered by the Nazis and all but my father's brother met the same fate. Yet family celebrations and the feasts of Jewish holidays were full of adults I called Aunty and Uncle. In truth, they were mostly distant cousins or unrelated friends, but they filled the house. I assumed I would always know them and their children, that we would always be connected.

When my mother died, though, at the age of sixty-three, contact dwindled and then stopped. She had been the social engine keeping us together, and the connections I had thought were muscle and blood, turned out to be flaky as skin.

73

My father moved to New York some years after my mother died. Although I am in regular contact with him by phone, neither of us has been able to travel for a while, and it is years since I have seen him face-to-face. And the only other member of the family I grew up with is my older sister.

Ours is a relationship that has always been difficult. She was a doted-on only child for the nearly four years before my birth and, for her, my arrival in the family came as that of a hated intruder. This remained the core of her relationship with me and was something I failed to understand throughout my childhood and adolescence. I only knew that no matter what I did to try to please her or win approval, I was met on a daily basis with malevolence and attack. I was a young adult before I freed myself from the cycle. It is nineteen years since she has spoken to me and I have long since accepted that this is how it will remain. There is an enormous sadness in siblings being estranged, but it is a painfully common experience.

Too many people have nodded their heads at the old saying 'Family is what you're given, friends are the ones you choose'. I am lucky in having some wonderful close and loving friends. All, however, lead 21st-century lives – ridiculously busy and juggling impossible schedules of work and family.

Since Martin's stroke, with me having to split most of my daylight hours between patients and being with Martin, my regular contacts with friends are mostly through hurried phone calls or emails, crammed into a narrow window of opportunity. When we succeed in meeting face to face, it is nourishingly wonderful, but those times are not frequent, although they are what I thirst for. I dream about a place where friends live within walking distance and time is available. Where neighbours are known and there is a community to act as extended family.

The first two weeks have been warmed by a comfort of support – friends dropping off food, phoning, emailing, texting. I notice a shift once that first fortnight has passed. The phone calls dwindle. The responses to my daily group email updates fall away. Whereas previously I might have had a dozen replies to my daily updates, now I might get only a couple.

A dropping-off is natural, of course, as people return to their everyday lives. The initial sense of shock and crisis is over. And many people are also unsure what to say as the difficult news drags on. What to say is in fact simple. Something as short as 'Thinking of you' or 'Sending love' is enough. What counts is the sense that you are responding, that you care, that the person is not forgotten.

One exception to the 'responding is good' rule comes with a correspondent who is relentlessly upbeat and positive about everything. Absolutely everything. Whatever the dire happenings that make their way onto the daily update, he will find a positive spin to them. As the weeks go on, these spins become both increasingly acrobatic and increasingly irksome. I fight the temptation to send a fake update to him, reporting that Martin has been knocked over and lost an arm and a leg. I feel convinced that the response would come back – 'Fantastic! He's got one arm and one leg left'. Eventually, I simply leave Mr Pollyanna off the update list, undoubtedly to our mutual relief.

I am also being introduced at an accelerated rate to the strange magic of modern communication technology. As in all the best fairytales, it involves both blessings and curses. The blessing is the mysterious ability to make writing appear on distant surfaces, thousands of miles or three feet away, instantaneously, effortlessly and with little expenditure of time or energy. The curse is the ability to make writing appear on distant surfaces, thousands of miles or three feet away, instantaneously, effortlessly and with little expenditure of time or energy.

We can send our thoughts to distant countries with a single press of the 'send' button. We can communicate by writing a message on a wall that will be instantly visible to anyone we wish at whatever time we send it. We can 'talk' to people we have never met and we can meet people we will never talk to. We have perfected the spell – we can talk without using our voices.

This gift of instant, voiceless communication is the most powerful magic, but like all magic, it extracts a cost. It is the spell made famous in Walt Disney's *Fantasia*. The film's most iconic scene is based on an ancient fairytale reimagined by Disney. In it, the lazy young magician's apprentice commands a broom to do the work he is supposed to do by hand – fetch buckets of water to fill a large water vat in the cavern. He loses control of the broom, it multiplies, and the many brooms relentlessly and unceasingly fetch, carry and pour the water so that the cavern becomes a raging sea and the young apprentice is thrown about at its mercy, at the point of drowning when he is rescued by the return of the magician.

Smart phones and iPads are everywhere. Most conversations these days are punctuated by taking calls, looking at messages, sending texts or tweets and catching up on the latest breaking fragment of 'news'. Attention is split between what is currently happening in the here and now, with the person you are with, and what might be happening elsewhere, with someone, or something, else. The gift of undiluted and uninterrupted attention is becoming a rarity. There is a generation growing up who may not know it. Studies are showing that even eye contact is becoming less frequent.

More and more, we are experiencing life with the kind of fractured attention that misses connections, emotions, subtleties and lacks the ability to follow through – all essential components of meaningful human connection. And we are also increasingly experiencing it at a distance. The phone answering machine, originally developed so that we would not miss those who called to talk to us, is now mostly used as a screening device so that we can avoid those who wish to speak to us. Emails, texting and instant messaging extend this distancing even further by requiring fewer words and eliminating the possibility of accidentally catching someone at home if you ring to leave a phone message.

Furthermore, when communication is focused on the screen, it bypasses the human voice. The voice is an instrument of supreme complexity. Emotions of the finest shades are layered into it through intonation, volume, pitch and rhythm. It is exquisitely expressive and responsive in both intentional and unintentional ways. It reveals the subtleties of the speaker's own emotional state as well as those in the messages it conveys. And the voice can only truly be experienced in the back-and-forth of real-time conversation. And so, even as I value the emails, texts and the people behind them, I miss their voices and the immediate, responsive and human connection they offer.

I am discovering, too, that even with the reduced requirements of emails and texts, some people cannot manage even the simple three- or four-word response these means of communication make so easy. Is it because these people are too fragile? Too busy? Uninterested? It is impossible to know, but their absence becomes highlighted simply because technology makes that brief reply so easy and economical that the act of withholding can speak loudly.

And there is also the reverse experience. Some months down the track, Miriam, an old friend, emails to say hello and to catch up. I email back and fill her in on what has been happening. She replies immediately, asking if I want to meet for a cup of coffee. It is so exactly what I need – matching what I have not voiced with the precision of a mind-reading trick – that I am unutterably moved. This offer – of time, coffee and a hug – made so naturally and spontaneously, is the magic gift.

I am very aware as I write my regular updates that no one wants to be confronted daily with dismal news. Although I write about Martin's ongoing medical experiences, I also take care to make the emails lively, readable, laced with humour. They become a kind of performance piece that says 'Keep interested. Keep reading. Keep connected'. There is only so much grimness people can bear, so I tap-dance my way between sharing Martin's progress, which is slow and uncertain, and enacting Scheherazade's ancient role. People tell me they look forward to the daily updates, enjoy reading them. On the one day I don't send one out, several people contact me, alarmed at the absence of the daily missive.

The updates are public pieces and there is an exterior quality to them. Everything contained in them is true, but my interior life is invisible. I don't write about sadness or the gripping terror that sometimes takes hold of me at thoughts of the possible future. I write about the day's doings, Martin's experiences, the medical system — it is a constructed narrative with the reader in mind. Nevertheless, writing these updates each day is nourishing in a way that is paradoxically hard to put into words. I am invariably exhausted but I miss only one day in two months of updates. As I sit writing them at the computer, I am talking to someone and it is not myself. Or rather, I am conversing with myself but also another. And as I do so, I am creating something, forming a story, making a connection. The Danish writer Isak Dinesen wrote that 'All sorrows can be borne if you put them in a story'. Perhaps it is not so much putting them in a story — they already are a story after all — but finding the right story to wrap around them.

We are born seeking stories. More than just wanting them, we need them. The human brain is hardwired to extract meaning from its environment. We look for causality, connection, the ways events or people relate to each other — all the things that make up a story. Our feelings and actions depend on which story we currently understand ourselves to be a part of. And which role we play in it. We are made of stories — that is what memories are, whether they be true or false. There are stories all around us — we are selective about which ones we pick out. And that in itself is a story.

I fell in love with words early. I was writing poems in preschool, reading whatever I could and entranced by written language. If there was nothing else to read, I would read the cereal boxes at the breakfast table. I insisted on learning the piano in primary school simply because I couldn't stand the idea that there was a system of notation I couldn't read. I read all about the lives of the great composers when I was seven. I devoured books about them. I knew every detail of their lives. And it never once occurred to me to listen to their music. I just wanted to know their stories. And stories were inextricably tied up with words.

Some years ago, as I wrote *Eating the Underworld*, the memoir of my journey through cancer, I found myself writing a section of it in the form of short stories exploring meaning in the world of fairy tale and folklore. The short story was a form I had never been drawn to previously, but felt compelled to use at this particular time. To say that I allowed myself to go with the flow would be inaccurate. Surprised as I was by what was coming out of my pen, I had no choice. Those stories wanted to write me.

Years later, I read that psychoanalysts have speculated that as stresses change in an illness trajectory, the means by which some artists express themselves also changes. It is as if the transformative task of creating must change itself in order to meet the changing destructive challenges of life-threatening illness. I gasped with recognition.

During the years of my cancer diagnosis and recurrence, what I needed to write and the style in which I needed to write it shifted sharply through the different stages – poetry, journal, short fiction – each refusing to be written in any other shape. Now, too, I am allowing myself to be chosen by the style of writing. Right now what I need to write comes in the form of these group updates – a genre in which I have never written before, never been interested in writing before. But here it is.

I am also starting to experience by now some of the paradoxes of being a carer. People are visiting Martin. He is the patient, the one people want to cheer up and remind that they care. It is natural for them to want to support the patient. The paradox lies in the fact that the patient is the one who is already being supported. He has the carer to support him and the professionals in the health system in whatever form they take. It is the carer in fact who needs support, often far more so than the patient. The carer is caring for the patient but no one is caring for the carer. I have certainly read about this – it is well documented, but for the first time I am experiencing it in vivo.

I have now lived both roles – I have been the patient, diagnosed with life-threatening illness and given an educated guess of two years to live. And I have been a carer. And being the patient was easier by far.

My friend Davida has also experienced both roles. Davida and I met in a cherished piece of serendipity. She was visiting Australia from her home in California. She had survived ovarian cancer and someone from the ovarian cancer discussion list told her of another survivor, a woman who lived in Melbourne, the city she was visiting. She contacted me and we met for coffee. When Davida told me that within days of arriving in Australia she had rented a car and driven herself down the Great Ocean Road, I was instantly impressed. And my first impressions were borne out. Davida is a very special person. We formed an immediate bond and have been dear friends ever since.

More than a decade ago, Davida nursed her husband through a terminal illness and then a few months later was diagnosed herself with ovarian cancer. I ask Davida which role she found harder, the patient diagnosed with cancer or the carer of a loved one suffering from a grave and uncertain illness. She answers without hesitation. Like me, she found the role of patient an easier one than that of carer.

'Why?' I ask her.

'The powerlessness', she responds.

And it is true that the carer often feels a tremendous sense of powerlessness. They have to watch the suffering of someone they love. It is often easier to experience the pain of treatments oneself than to watch helplessly as they are administered. That is certainly true for me, but it is not the total explanation.

I turn the question over in my mind. My answer is still clear but the whys and wherefores are harder to pin down. Fatigue, loneliness and fear – all three are equally familiar to both the carer and patient. But they are experienced differently. When I was twice diagnosed with a deadly cancer, it was frightening but it had a different edge. I didn't want to die, but the urgency of that need to stay alive was very much to do with the fact that my daughter was a teenager – it was unbearable to think of the devastating impact my death would have on her. For myself, although I wanted very much to stay alive, I was not frightened of my death. I had no trouble envisaging it – one day I would simply wink into non-existence. I wouldn't be there to know about it.

As a carer, though, if the worst happens, I am acutely aware that I will be there to know about it. And that is the extra factor – I am afraid of that pain, of the terrible grief that will need to be moved through. I have experienced death before. I nursed my mother, whom I loved dearly, through the final months of her illness. She died too young and I still miss her, but in a sense we expect our parents to die. It is part of the natural order of things. It feels utterly different when imagining the death of a life partner.

In *A Grief Observed*, C. S. Lewis, a theologian as well as the author of the *The Lion, the Witch and the Wardrobe*, wrote about the experience of losing his beloved wife Joy: 'No one ever told me that grief felt so like fear...'

Joan Didion, who suffered the intolerable double blow of having both her husband and daughter die within a short time of each other, wrote in her memoir *Blue Nights*, 'I was no longer, if I had ever been, afraid to die: I was now afraid not to die'.

Their words resonate deeply. I have been lucky so far. Martin is alive. But this is where I go in the worst of imagined futures.

25 June 2009

The physio has been noticing some signs of movement in Martin's shoulder, an encouraging sign, as the paralysis of his arm has up to now been stubbornly resistant. His OT time has been focused on learning to do things one-handed. When I sat in on his class a few days ago, I watched with admiration as he tried again and again to master the trick of doing up shoelaces one-handed until finally he succeeded. The number of small, essential daily tasks for which we so automatically assume the use of two hands is mind-boggling. Each one of them represents an Everest for Martin. I wonder to myself whether I would have been able to persevere with such patience and determination had I been in his situation. I sadly suspect that the answer is no.

Martin's speech now has several words that can be made out clearly and he is better able to write down the word he is trying to say. He has to write, of course, with his left hand but more than the inconvenience of this, it takes enormous effort for him to find the right letters to denote whatever word he is thinking of. He cannot usually manage more than one word, and the effort of trying to get the word in his head to become the word on the page is tremendous – you can see it in his expression and the tension in his whole body, but at least he is beginning to manage it some of the time.

I ask him whether he thinks a lot about things, as in Life, the Universe, what has happened to him and so on, and he shakes his head and writes the word 'jumbled'. It seems the perfect choice to describe the inner workings of Martin's mind at this stage, with so much to relearn and make sense of. It is also wonderful to know that within the jumble, he has been able to locate and express the precise word that describes its interior, blurry home.

This morning I am sitting in on another of Martin's speech therapy sessions. Today the therapist is trying to teach Martin how to form the sound 'p'. Martin's brain is completely at a loss as to how to do this – it has not the first notion of what instructions to give to the muscles of mouth and tongue. The speech therapist is helping Martin by showing him the shape her lips form as she pronounces the sound 'p' and how she expels her breath at the same time. Martin looks closely and you can see him straining, really straining as he attempts to reproduce the sound.

After several tries, he finally manages to produce an approximation of the sound.

'Great!' says the therapist. 'Now, do it again'.

And they do it again and again. Each time you can see how much work it requires of Martin. This simple, minuscule task, so effortless and trivial that it is effectively invisible in our day-to-day interactions, is the equivalent of running a triathlon for Martin's new brain. But he persists. And gradually I can see it is getting just slightly, slightly easier.

As the session finishes, the therapist remarks casually that Martin might be ready for weekend leave soon. Weekend leave! I hadn't even realised there was such a thing.

bathroom, his own armchair, his computer, the uninterrupted nights – all the home comforts that have been so drastically missing for him over the last weeks.

28 June 2009

Denise has invited us over today to celebrate my birthday. We tuck in to a second birthday cake and another successful round of the 'Happy Birthday' song. Martin cannot stop smiling.

Late this afternoon, I pack Martin's bags and take him back to the hospital. After stowing his belongings back in the hospital locker and bedside drawers, Martin settles back in his bedside chair with a smile. I ask him what he is thinking and he says four words slowly but distinctly – 'I feel so content'.

Even though Martin was only back home for one night, tonight the house feels once again resonant with his absence. I sit down and make a list of what I have to do tomorrow. It includes chasing up the time of Martin's appointment at Prince Edward for an MRI of his brain.

Martin's MRI appointment was originally supposed to be next week. Then there was a phone call saying it had been shifted to this Thursday. Following that, a letter arrived telling me that it was indeed this week, but at a different time from the one previously mentioned. This was followed by another phone message citing an appointment next week on a different day. Trying not to feel like a contestant on an obscure game show, I ring the Prince Edward to ascertain which is correct. After much checking of appointment lists, consulting with mysterious others and undoubtedly the throwing and interpretation of burnt chicken bones, the receptionist comes back to tell me that yes, the appointment is this Thursday. I plan to ring again tomorrow to confirm that the wandering appointment has indeed lost momentum and is fixed to the one spot.

30 June 2009

Martin continues to make progress day by day. It is slow but discernible – more noticeable to those who see him less regularly than to the everyday visitor, but even the minutest change is noted by me. Every change, no matter how fractional, is cause for hope.

And in an exciting development, Trevor is no longer resident at South-Central. He has been moved to the Prince Edward. A youngish man occupies his bed and is extraordinary in that he seems reasonable, quite smart and pleasant. Sadly for us and luckily for him, he will be moving out next week. Costas is still reclining and declaiming (loudly) about all manner of things in his stolen best bed. The nurses are chocolate-free.

I am re-reading *My Year Off*, a memoir by Robert McCrum, a well-known writer and editor who, at the age of forty-two, woke one morning to discover he had suffered a massive stroke. I read it when it was first published in 1998 but have taken it down from the shelf again.

What I remember from my first reading was a beautifully written, if harrowing, memoir. But what grabs me this time is something different. Alternating with McCrum's voice is that of his newlywed wife, Sarah Lyall. It is her story I am drawn to this time. And when, in one brief section early on, she describes her concern about how she will cope if her husband doesn't recover, I am glued to the page. Her words are like water on a dry day. Right now I don't want to read about heroism or altruism or any of those pure or virtuous words – I want to read about fear, about the murky side of uncertainty, about someone who is scared witless, who doesn't know if she is up for it, or even what she is up for except that it could be terrifyingly beyond her capacity.

That is the horror-stricken part of myself I don't attend to but I know is there, the one that knows the future could be impossibly grim. Right now it is hope that has to power me, and as long as Martin is making progress, be it halting or slow, I can take that ride. It is only when it stops that I will have to find out where I am and what I am made of. Robert McCrum makes a good recovery and Sarah Lyall makes only that one reference to her own doubts about what she is capable of, but I love her for it.

I am reading every memoir I can lay my hands on about a partner being plunged into catastrophic illness. They are frightening, but I am prepared to be frightened. It is the price I pay for discovering how people cope, and I search them out avidly. I don't know anyone else in my position. I have made some attempts to find a support group for partners of those who are in the same phase of recovery as Martin, but either they don't exist or my search techniques are inadequate. Memoirs become my only way of spending time with a fellow traveller.

1 July 2009

Martin continues to work assiduously on his speech. His speech therapy sessions take up an hour or so each day, but in between he has speech homework – pages of word-matching puzzles, sentence-completion tasks and the like. He can write a greater number of words now, and his spoken vocabulary is growing a little each day – he can now put a few words together into phrases.

The effort he has to make to pronounce these words is clear. Each word is spoken with the care and slow precision of a non-native speaker who is learning English from a spoken-word disc. The spoken-word disc Martin has in his head is narrated by an educated Englishman. It is not that of Martin's natural accent.

The Australian accent is considered to fall into three main groups – broad, general and cultivated. Broad is the more extreme accent associated with pure 'Strine', general is less nasal but nevertheless distinctly Australian, and cultivated is closer to what we think of as an English accent. Martin, like me and almost all of our friends, has a general Australian accent. Now the operative tense, however, is 'had'. Martin's old accent, the one in which he voiced his thoughts for all of his speaking years, has vanished.

It is not only the accent that has changed. Something else has changed. Writers commonly talk of finding the 'voice' of their characters. They mean not only the words the characters utter but the tone in which they are spoken: the ways these words, which lie silent on a page, take on a timbre, an intonation that colours in for us the character of the speaker. This unquantifiable yet definite character of Martin's speech has changed, as well as his accent. There is a flatness to his speech, which is technically termed 'robotic', and it does indeed have the characteristic of robotic recorded responses in which each word is equally accented without the natural lift and fall of our normal speaking voices. But equally striking is a quality almost the opposite to that of the robot. It is the quality of a child learning to speak.

There is a new vulnerability in Martin's voice. I am reminded of a young child struggling to comprehend the vastness of an alphabet, the enormous mountain ranges of words and the importance, and impossibility, of not just choosing, but pronouncing, the one correct, exact sound in all of those hundreds of sounds. Impossibly difficult. But the child is trying anyway.

This vulnerability, a sort of gentle earnestness that acknowledges struggle and weakness without defensiveness, is something I have never seen in Martin. Martin has always been a high achiever. Always able to do whatever he set his hand to. Effortlessly topping his classes throughout his school and university years, single-handedly changing his Volvo from a manual to an automatic, mastering any number of crafts and skills. He is used to being in control, to being on top of things, to learning things with speed and ease. He is a generous person but doesn't tolerate fools easily, and that includes himself when he makes mistakes. He is not especially patient with the slow. He is used to having energy and being organised, and finds it hard to understand those who are not. He is used to being, in other words, exactly the opposite of the person he is now.

And the person he is now feels different in other ways as well. There is a shift not just in the sense of his gentleness, but in other aspects that are equally hard to quantify. He is more affectionate, more patient, more empathic. Whereas previously Martin has always assumed I could take care of myself, now he wants to reach out and take care of me. Qualities he took for granted in me, he now appreciates. The transformation is both wonderful and strange.

Changes like this are the opposite of those usually connected to stroke or brain damage. Volatility, impulsiveness and temper tantrums are much more common accompaniments – caused by the destruction of parts of the brain associated with self-control, planning and reasoning. I haven't heard of the opposite happening. Are these new aspects of Martin just a grateful reaction to surviving a life-threatening crisis? A result of forced dependency? Something that will revert if or when life gets back to an approximation of normal? I don't know and I tend to suspect the latter. Martin's personality is Martin's personality, after all – it has been fixed for decades. It is different from his intellectual and cognitive abilities. I can understand those shifting with injury to his brain. These other characteristics – this new tenderness, this new empathic caring – are so much more than cognitive skills, they are core aspects of personality, of relationship. It seems astonishing that they could suddenly change in such a deep way.

And yet…I have been reading to Martin from *My Stroke of Insight*, the extraordinary memoir by Jill Bolte Taylor, a young neuroscientist who suffered a massive bleed in her brain in much the same area as Martin's. She describes her left hemisphere dropping out as the bleed in it progressed. With it went linear, logical, speech-oriented thinking. At the same time, however, Bolte Taylor writes that she also experienced her right hemisphere, now unrestrained by left-hemisphere influence, taking over, an experience she describes as spiritual – a consciousness liberated from physical boundaries – and timeless.

Clearly, both hemispheres are needed in order to survive, and Bolte Taylor has to struggle to understand what numbers are as she makes difficult and prolonged attempts to dial for help. By the time she reaches hospital she has lost all ability to speak and understand speech, has lost numeracy, has lost the ability to understand causal logical sequences (such as the need to put socks on before shoes instead of vice versa) and much else. She makes an extraordinary recovery over the next few years, regaining fluency and speech comprehension to the extent that she is now an eloquent and polished speaker who has authored a beautifully written and best-selling memoir. Within this account of her recovery, she describes emerging with a changed personality, one that differs from her previous type-A persona. She describes herself as more compassionate, more peaceful and loving. When I read this section to Martin, he nods with recognition. 'Yes', he says. 'I understand'.

2 July 2009

This morning as I enter the ward a nurse catches me with the news that Martin is to be shifted to another ward. And, amazingly enough, it is the good ward I first spotted on his arrival at South-Central – a three-bed ward that actually has quiet, pleasant occupants.

There was a happy confluence of events that dictated this result. The two occupants of Martin's new ward had previously had a very loud, very disturbed third person in the bed now to be occupied by Martin. They combined to protest vehemently, saying they would not tolerate this and needed to have someone quieter for their ward. Their protest and my pleadings for Martin to move to a more peaceful ward created a perfect synergy of requests/demands and so the loud troublemaker was moved out and Martin is to be moved in.

As Martin's bed is wheeled in, two rather white-faced occupants of the new ward look at me and demand anxiously to know if Martin is 'quiet'. I assure them that he is and restrain myself from adding that in fact he can barely speak, and we all settle down in harmony.

Although the physios have been noting that there is now some movement in Martin's shoulder and that with some effort, he can now move his arm upwards against gravity, his hand remains paralysed and essentially useless. It seems his progress in this area is slower than it should be. Last night, however, I had an interesting thought.

Back in the far-off days before Martin's stroke, I had been reading about the treatment of phantom limb pain through mirror boxes. Phantom limb pain – pain felt in an absent, amputated limb – has been notoriously difficult to treat. In 1998, however, one of the most brilliant neuroscientists of modern times, V. S.

Ramachandran, theorised that phantom limb pain was the result of the brain being 'stuck' on the last recorded sensations from that limb before amputation, so that even though the actual limb was no longer there, the brain was still reacting as though it was present and in its painful, unpleasant pre-surgery state. He reasoned that if the brain could be fooled into thinking it was receiving 'normal' messages from the limb, the pain might disappear.

To this end he devised a simple contraption called a mirror box. The patient would use their good hand to pick up small objects while looking into a mirror set at an angle. Because of the mirror's reflection, it would look as if it was in fact the opposite (amputated) hand that was moving the objects and thus fool the brain into thinking it was receiving normal and pain-free signals from the amputated hand. Ramachandran obtained excellent results with his mirror box.

The same principle, it would seem, can be applied to a hand that has been paralysed through stroke. The brain tends to operate on a 'Use it or lose it' principle. If the neurons relating to the movement of a right hand, for example, stop firing because the hand is paralysed, it can become a vicious circle. The less the hand moves, the less stimulated the neurons are, and the less stimulated the neurons, the less the hand moves, and so on. If the brain is fooled through the mirror box into thinking the paralysed right hand is moving, it may stimulate the neurons and they in turn might actually help the hand to move.

More research is still needed in the area and explanations and results differ, but it definitely seems worth a try. I get onto the computer and within minutes have ordered my very own mirror box. It arrives with amazing speed within two days, and I bring it to Martin's physio session. We set it up and Martin starts to carry out some simple tasks with his good left hand while gazing into the mirror, so that it looks as if it is his right hand doing the work.

The first thing he notices is that his left hand feels strangely heavy and awkward. This sounds promising, as if something more than just picking up objects with a perfectly functional hand is occurring. By the next day, Martin is reporting the occasional odd sensation in his paralysed right hand, as if it is just about to move, and within just a few more days, his right hand is starting to have movement. The excitement is enormous – it is not a controlled double-blind study, but we are all willing to bet that it was the mirror box that did it.

For Martin, the relief of seeing progress in his hand is greater than that of seeing progress in his speech. He has grown up building things, fixing things, working with his hands, and the thought of being left effectively one-handed is horrifying to him. From that first twitch of movement, he works diligently at his assigned tasks. Over the next couple of weeks, the results are reported with jubilation – he can lift a spoon, he can manipulate a fork, he can shakily write a word – the paralysis is fading with each day.

3 July 2009

Charles had ordered another MRI at the Prince Edward more than a week ago. Its purpose was to continue the hunt for any vascular deformities that might explain Martin's stroke and may or may not require neurosurgery if found. The other purpose was to look at the level of residual post-stroke damage now that a month has passed.

The results were supposed to have been sent back by the Prince Edward to South-Central days ago. I have been up and down the rabbit hole continuously ever since attempting to find someone who a) has them, and b) will tell me about them.

Finally, this morning Charles manages to locate both the MRI and the associated report. The good news is there is no vascular deformity and therefore no brain surgery is required. However, as Charles puts it, the MRI also shows that there is a blood clot the size of a golf ball in there. He shows us the actual scan and we gulp. There is Martin's brain and there within it is a giant black inkblot covering all of his expressive speech area and a bit more besides. The image, in all of its unambiguous blackness and vastness, is shocking to behold.

Although, realistically, it is simply the clotted bleed that showed up in the Frankston scan, which we had already been told covered a three by three by three-centimetre area, somehow we had both held onto the fantasy that it would have magically melted away. I ask Charles what will happen to that clot and he says it will dissolve over the course of a year or so but that the area where it had been will remain empty space – the brain cells within it are dead and will not revive.

The other aspect of the MRI is that with no vascular deformities showing up and the echocardiogram showing no heart problems, the 'why' question about the stroke remains unanswered. The doctors have now explored every explanatory avenue they can think of but no answers have presented themselves.

5 July 2009

Martin is enjoying his second weekend leave at home. Other than the obvious handicaps caused by the stroke, he is feeling well. He is walking strongly and his appetite is extremely healthy – he is having sumptuous three-course meals for lunch and dinner, complete with dessert. And on this diet, read this and weep, Martin has lost two kilos. As has often been said, if we could patent Martin's metabolism, we could retire in luxury, buy several large islands, end world poverty and ace numerous other impossible financial goals.

Taking Martin back to hospital after weekend leave feels like taking a child back to a bleak boarding school after term holidays. There is a very Dickensian feel about the return to South-Central. To add to the illusion, Martin in fact travels with about as much luggage as a boarding school child – I have two bags in each hand and one hanging off either shoulder.

6 July 2009

Today is exactly a month since Martin's stroke. His progress has been wonderful. The speech therapists love working with him – changes are happening every day and they look forward to seeing him after each weekend to discover what new things he has been able to master over the two days they were absent from the centre.

Yesterday, as I walked back from picking something up at the chemist, I saw the light turn green just a few feet from where I was. To catch the green light, I would have to pick up my pace but much as I told my feet to move faster, they simply refused to obey. It was the most peculiar feeling. I am so used to my body doing, or at least attempting to do, what I tell it to that it seemed impossibly strange, like a phone line dropping out in the middle of an animated conversation. I could hear my internal orders going feet-wards but my muscles simply refused to respond and gave no explanation. I realised that in a minuscule way, this must be what Martin feels with his paralysed arm.

This evening I suspect I am running a temperature from a second bug I picked up more than a week ago. I know I should get the thermometer out and measure it, but I am too tired. I finished my patients at 7.00 pm and have been huddled under two blankets while wearing two jumpers and I am still shivering. Tomorrow, though, I have to get to South-Central first thing, as this is Charles's weekly round and it is the only opportunity to catch and question the otherwise elusive team.

Charles's junior medical proxy on a day-to-day basis is the medical resident Jane, otherwise known to us as Jane the Pain. She walks around with a thought bubble permanently affixed to her head reading 'Whatever…', with the full quota of adolescent scorn and dismissal attached to its unspoken syllables. Any question addressed to her invariably gets a response that can be summarised by this word. An opportunity to snare Charles instead of Jane is not to be missed.

By an intense effort of will, I haul myself to the bathroom to brush my teeth and then fall into bed. Just before collapsing into sleep, I ring Martin to say goodnight and manage to have a small but definitely intelligible conversation with him. Amazing!

7 July 2009

I wake up this morning bathed in sweat and feeling even more exhausted than the previous evening. I stagger to the bathroom and stare foggily at the apparition staring foggily back at me. My bedside literature over the last few days has been a book on the dancing plagues of the sixteenth century. Clearly my imagination has taken me too far into the mediaeval world of my reading material. I could swear those are pustules on my face.

A visit to the doctor brings the news that they are indeed pustules – I am in the process of beginning an encounter with the adult version of chickenpox. My first thought is about my state of infectiousness and the people with whom I have been in contact. This level of altruistic thinking is only possible in the very, very early stages of adult chickenpox. Once past day one, altruism flies out the window.

The GP, whom I have not seen before, informs me that no, I was not infectious yesterday when I saw my patients, as well as Martin and Amantha. And in response to my second question, he says no, there is no prophylactic treatment Amantha can take to prevent her coming down with it. I know that Martin has already had childhood chickenpox but, alarmingly, Amantha hasn't. Despite my foggy state, I feel sure that the GP is mistaken and that a) I was contagious yesterday, and b) some kind of prophylactic action is possible for Amantha.

I make enquiries of Dr Google but cannot seem to find the right answers. The friends I ring agree that my guesses feel intuitively right but can offer no hard information. And then Lynne, bless her heart, says 'Why not ask Nurse-On-Call. '

'Nurse-On-Call?' I echo.

And it turns out that our government, in an unusually splendid use of our tax dollars, has funded Nurse-On-Call – a 24/7 service where the nurse on call provides you with health information for any questions you might want to ask.

I speedily dial the appropriate number and am connected with a delightful nurse who confirms that yes, the infectious period for chickenpox is indeed a day or two before the pustules appear.

My next question – whether vaccination could be preventative if given within a window of time after exposure is not so speedily answered. The nurse searches for a while among various medical texts but cannot find anything. She suggests I ring the Immunisation Department and is just on the point of hanging up in order to allow me to do so, when she suddenly finds a paragraph at the back of a sheaf of papers stating that immunisation within three to five days of exposure may prevent or minimise the appearance of chickenpox post-exposure. In triumph, I ring Amantha immediately and send her off for said vaccination.

The next calls are to my patients of yesterday, who luckily have all had childhood chickenpox. Then phone calls to Martin and South-Central. And then I settle down to be sick. Really sick – with all the mediaeval splendour of head-to-toe pustules, drenching sweats and the thrill of the spit-over-your-shoulder, make-the-sign-of-the-evil-eye and keep-away-from-me-at-all-costs isolation of quarantine.

In response to my morning phone call, South-Central puts out an infection alert for Martin's unit, making me a shoo-in for the Miss Popularity contest. Luckily, as it turns out, the only person who seems to be susceptible to my brand of chickenpox is me.

Chickenpox in adults is not for chickens. The drenching sweats take me through four nighties a night. In the morning I have just enough energy to drop them in the washing machine and drop myself back onto the bed. My skin is so tender and painful that the only thing I can bear next to it is the softness of my oldest flannel nighties worn inside out so the seams don't feel like barbed wire against my skin. Everything else feels as if I am wearing a thorny hairshirt next to my skin in the manner of certain monks but without the resultant spiritual uplift. The only thing that brings a small temporary relief from the all-over aching and itching is my recommended Pinetarsol bath. These bright-yellow baths are the highlight of my day.

As the days go on, I am more wretchedly sick than at any other time in my life, and this includes chemotherapy and recoveries from major surgery. I am febrile, exhausted beyond belief and in constant pain. Yesterday, while staring in frustration at my stubbornly receding Pinetarsol bath, I discovered an important law of physics – the bath fills better when there is a plug in place. It took me fifteen minutes to work this out – the constant presence of fever, no sleep and whatever other havoc adult chickenpox wreaks on the brain is making its mark.

Update, 10 July 2009

Greetings from Chickenpox World. On my way upstairs to write this update, I happened to glance in the mirror. I immediately understood that the practice of quarantining the chickenpox sufferer has a twofold purpose. It is not just to prevent disease spreading, it is the equally imperative need to protect society from accidentally viewing the chickenpox face. With my heart barely recovering after its unexpected encounter with the ghoul in the mirror, I proceeded upstairs, telling myself that it was only me. How reassuring.

The chickenpox patient, I have been told, is considered infectious until the pustules start turning black and dropping off. My pustule-watch morning and night has brought no satisfaction – they are getting bigger but not blacker, and cover almost every visible inch of my skin and scalp. Washing my hair is out of the question because of the exquisitely painful pustules, and my hair is about ready to get up and walk by itself.

Every few days, Amantha drops a load of supermarket staples on the doorstep and backs off rapidly so as to avoid contagious contact, but apart from that, no other human comes near. As the days of enforced isolation have gone by, I have been craving the nourishment of simple face-to-face contact. There must be a niche market for adult sufferers of chickenpox – P&P parties: pyjamas and pustules.

I have ploughed on with my uncannily appropriate reading matter, however, and my in vivo peasant experience (filthy hair, pox, and so on) is adding flavour to the history of the dancing plagues. I have just enough brain power left to be grateful that the rest of the peasant experience – appalling housing, not enough food, excessive rodent population, and so on – is being gained in a less than in-vivo manner.

The timing of my reading material is also spot on (pun unintended) in other ways. This coming Tuesday, 14 July marks the anniversary of the beginning of the great dancing plague of 1518. On that day, Frau Troffea stepped outside her home in Strasbourg and began to dance without stopping, although bleeding and injured, for several days, thus beginning a deadly dancing epidemic that infected hundreds of people. At one stage of the epidemic, fifteen people were dying every day from the remorseless unstoppable dancing. Chroniclers of the time report that dancers often held hands and danced in circles. This at least is one thing chickenpox does not incline you to do.

On the good news side, Susan, Martin's speech pathologist, who is the liaison for the team, rang to tell me the results of yesterday's team meeting. To summarise – they are thrilled with Martin's progress. They love having Martin as their patient – she said he does them good. And she told me Martin can now pick up a cup. Martin's release date is currently early August, so they are planning on giving him lots of intensive work as an inpatient because he is responding so well.

Anyway, off to apply calamine lotion.

12 July 2009

I have been hoping against hope that the pustules will oblige by retreating in time for me to be with Martin on his 15 July birthday. The pustules, however, have no such goal in mind. They remain stubbornly thriving and in a state of health inverse to mine.

They cover almost every inch of skin and, with my lank, stringy hair, I could make money hiring myself out to mediaeval fairs to bring that touch of authenticity to the proceedings. I am definitely a sight to make eyes sore. This morning, while I was gloomily inspecting the pustules covering my face, the phone rang. 'Is this the Looking Good Display Centre?' said the voice on the other end.

Einstein forgot to include adult chickenpox in his discussion of the relativity of time. Six days have crawled by and I am still waiting for those damn pustules to turn black and indicate that I am no longer infectious and can do things like walk in the street and, pinnacle of excitement, go to the supermarket. In contrast, when I rang Martin this afternoon to see how he was, he said rather rapidly, 'Rushed off my feet. Physio got put up to one o'clock. Had to hurry to eat my lunch. Call you later'.

Martin's speech has come on so well that he can now sustain a ten-minute conversation with me. We speak mostly in the evenings, when he has finished his program for the day, and it is amazing to think that just over a month ago he was incapable of making even a sound – and now we are having a conversation.

Martin is currently outfitted with a 24-hour cardiac monitor to see how his heart is functioning (the doctors are still searching for the causes that might be behind the stroke). As well as going through his normal daily activities with the heart monitor on, they had Martin pedal for a stretch on an exercise bike to see how his heart did under stress. There was also an unplanned stress test in the evening as Martin took on the challenge of talking me through the process of recording TV programs. Given Martin's predilection for gadgets, we have no less than four separate remote controls for our TV and DVD-recorder. In the days when we had two controls, I had (just) been able to manage the recording and viewing process. By four controls I had well and truly given up. Martin managed this feat of techno-education, by distance and with a limited vocabulary, admirably and, to everyone's amazement, I successfully recorded a TV program.

13 July 2009

The pustules are still continuing to get bigger but not blacker. Martin, too, is continuing to make amazing progress. He actually managed a half-hour conversation with me this morning and told me he can now touch his right thumb to each of his opposing fingers, something he couldn't do last night. He mentions that his head is feeling clearer as well, and that he can speak in sentences and convey his thoughts in more complex ways than the simple one-word responses he was limited to less than two weeks ago. His voice is still mechanical, without the natural fluidity and shades of tone we take for granted and, interestingly, he cannot hear the difference between this and his natural pre-stroke voice.

Yesterday evening I was on the phone with Martin reading to him about the work of Taub (a pioneer in brain plasticity) on constraint therapy with stroke patients. This involves constraining the good arm, thereby forcing the affected arm to take its place in whatever small ways it can. The constant forced practice thus achieved seems to revive the 'brain map' of the affected arm. Taub has been getting terrific results through this method. This morning I learned that the physio and OT are so pleased with Martin they are thinking of starting him on constraint therapy in a week or two. Martin is very excited at this news.

Martin is, in fact, much chirpier than I am. Certainly much busier. He is on a very full schedule this week – three hours of physio today, for instance – and is only free for an hour at lunchtimes. In previous weeks he would have gaps of three hours when I could take him home for lunch. He is continuing to make improvements day by day and today he held a biro in his right hand and did some rudimentary writing.

Hearing of his exploits, I am reminded of those time-lapse videos of flower buds unfolding. It is as if the changes happen overnight. I imagine his brain as he sleeps, with its connections being reformed, repositioned and reaching out to each other in the manner of petals unfurling.

I think back now to those two stretched-out weeks following his stroke when he was unable to sound even a consonant, let alone form a single word, and the predictions of his treating professionals were uniformly gloomy. I remember searching for stories of people recovering from stroke, desperately trying to find the story that let me say 'If they can do it, so can you'.

Jill Bolte Taylor's extraordinary account of her recovery from a devastating stroke was a blaze of light in that grim firmament, as was Norman Doidge's *The Brain That Changes Itself.* They were the stories I fuelled myself with, the stories I told Martin about over and over. I thank whatever governs fate that they were in existence for me when I needed them so very much.

Despite all the repeated investigations, no one has yet been able to find a cause for Martin's stroke. The silver lining of that cloud is that the investigations are uniformly continuing to come back as normal. His heart looks to be in good working order, there are no malformed blood vessels to be seen in his brain or the arteries leading up to it. I tell myself this is good news, that it means he is essentially healthy. The stroke may remain forever mysterious, but it will be a one-off and he will recover from it. It feels as if we have crossed the mountain, managed to avoid the precipice and are now cruising downhill. Martin has only two weeks to go at South-Central and then he will be home. He may not be functioning in exactly the way he was pre-stroke, but he is doing so well that I feel confident he will be functioning competently – able to speak, walk and use his right hand. I know the kinds of exercise and training he needs to keep progress continuing and it is all manageable. It is all in sight – we are on the way to being home free.

14 July 2009

Tomorrow is Martin's birthday and for the first time I see signs that my pustules are relenting. I will be forced to remain in quarantine for his birthday but am hoping it will be safe to be back in the world by the weekend. It will be the first birthday in thirty-seven years we have spent apart. Which makes it nearly four decades since we met…

It is 1973. You are a girl with a problem. The boy you think you are going out with lives in Melbourne, as do you. The boy you really like is in Sydney. He is coming to Melbourne this weekend for a visit. What do you do with your Melbourne boy? Introduce him to the friend of a friend on a Thursday and pick him up again on the Monday when the Sydney boy is gone? Yes? No?

It is early evening on Thursday at my house. A girlfriend is keeping me company while I go through the process of defuzzing my underarms. The tool at hand is a tube of disgusting cream misleadingly labelled Veet-O. The O stands for odourless, which it is not.

I am halfway through the process, which involves waiting for an interminably long time while the Veet-O acts as the equivalent of Agent Orange for underarm hair. It is a process I hate but feel inadequate to protest against – the days of proud hairy armpits are yet to come and are due, of course, to vanish again decades later as the Brazilian rises up to demand even more cultural servility.

I am standing in the slightly awkward posture required of this process – arms raised in the air in the 'surrender' position, chatting to my friend when the doorbell rings.

I vaguely wonder who has come to visit my parents. I am not expecting anyone.

My mother pokes her head around the bathroom door. 'Your friend has come to visit you', she says to Hannah.

Hannah and I turn to each other. What friend? And why is Hannah's friend visiting her at my place?

I send Hannah off to entertain the mysterious visitors while I mutter grimly to myself as I check an armpit in the vain hope that the Veet-O has had time to work. No, of course it hasn't. And now I have to wash the whole mess off, entertain my unwanted visitors and repeat the Veet-O experience as soon as they leave. I am not a happy camper.

After attempting to rearrange the expression on my face, there is nothing for it but to go out and greet my visitors.

I can hear some voices as I walk down the corridor – Hannah, her friend and her friend's friend, who is a boy. He is sitting in a big armchair with his back to me – I can just see the top of his head.

And at that moment, as I walk towards him, his face still invisible to me, a voice in my head says, quite distinctly, 'You're going to marry him'. The voice is clear, concise and masculine. And it is definitely in my head.

To say I am startled is an understatement. I am at a time in my life when I am not looking for a boyfriend. I am in love with my new profession – I am learning how to be a psychotherapist; I am writing poetry in a whole new way and getting close to being published; I am doing an almost full-time clinical internship at a psychiatric hospital and, as well as that, I have to write a full-length dissertation for my masters degree in my 'spare' time. I have my hands well and truly full and I am loving it.

In addition to that, although recent research has shown that a very large number of normal people regularly hear voices in their head, I am not used to vocal accompaniments, particularly masculine ones, proclaiming anything except my own known thoughts.

I walk on and the resident of the armchair rises to greet me along with the two girls. He is a nice-looking boy. Glasses. Slightly built. A pleasant, intelligent face. Nothing that jumps out at me. I have no idea why some disembodied entity thinks I should be marrying him. It is certainly not in my plans.

I make the requisite cups of tea and coffee and we all start chatting. I have just finished reading *I Never Promised You a Rose Garden* by Joanne Greenberg. It is the gripping, semi-autobiographical novel of a teenage girl's years in the terrifying world of severe mental illness. I have been blown away by the book and extol its virtues rhapsodically. Martin is an engineer. He likes reading science fiction and detective novels. Full stop. He expresses a keen interest in reading *I Never Promised You a Rose Garden*. I lend it to him. And after a couple of hours of coffee and chat, the visit ends.

The next evening at 6.00 pm, the doorbell rings. Martin is standing there with my copy of *I Never Promised You a Rose Garden*, which he has spent the day reading. I am impressed.

We sit at the kitchen table with coffee and talk. At 3.00 am, we are still talking. One of us has just looked at the clock and realised what the time is and we have just risen from the kitchen table and are standing at the front door talking. At 6.00 am we are still standing at the door talking.

The next day, Martin comes over for a visit and stays through the evening. And repeats his visit the next day and the next day. This has never happened before to either of us.

I have a dilemma. I don't want to get into a steady relationship right now. I have been sent four highly prized invitations to the opening of a glamorous new discotheque in town – I could invite Martin or I could invite someone else. I make a deliberate decision. I am not going to invite Martin to go with me. I ask another boy instead. And the remaining two invitations I give to Hannah.

I arrive at the opening and go to the table, which Hannah, who was to arrive before me, will be keeping for me. Except that it is not Hannah who is sitting at the table, it is Martin. He has realised that I will be there and wangled the invite. At this point I give up.

Every evening after coming home from working at the hospital, I head for the dining-room table where the bits and pieces of my thesis-to-be are laid out. Every evening, just as I sit down, there is a ring on the doorbell. Martin has arrived.

Martin is doing a masters in electrical engineering. He is getting close to the end of his thesis. I started my masters degree in clinical psychology a year later than Martin. I am only in the middle of my thesis. We regularly have conversations in which we both agree that I do need to work on my thesis and that Martin doesn't need to be here every night. But every evening there is the ring on the doorbell. And every evening I am glad to hear it.

Within two weeks of meeting each other, we both know that we are going to marry each other. It is not said aloud but the understanding is so mutual and so clear that neither of us can recall the occasion of a proposal. It was never a question of if we would get married, it was simply a matter of deciding when. And that 'when' was a year after we had first met.

It is months after that first meeting that I get to hear about the motivation behind it – that Hannah's friend brought Martin over to my place with the idea of 'lending' him out for a few days. Martin is as startled as I am – he had thought of Hannah's friend only as a friend, not as a girlfriend. It was a crazily quirky plan, but we are both very glad of it.

Socrates has said that love is a sort of madness, although a madness that is a gift given by the gods. The experience of falling in love sets off a neurological cocktail involving oxytocin, vasopressin, dopamine, serotonergic signalling and the activation of endorphins, endogenous morphinergic systems and nitric oxide autoregulatory pathways, as well as a host of other complex neurobiological systems. These changes have been said to resemble those observed in people with substance abuse and psychosis.

In Martin's case they have had the remarkable effect of turning on his need to talk. A couple of years down the track, when we have settled happily into the 'in love' stage as opposed to the 'falling' stage, Martin's brain settles down to its normal Martin level. 'Chat', 'talk' and 'converse' are words that rarely pop their heads above Martin's horizon. He is the archetypal man of few words, something that becomes deeply ironic in the present, as words and their production become the main focus of his days.

To some outsiders we may seem like an odd coupling: Martin is interested in objects, I am interested in people. Martin is practical and unsentimental, I am creative and definitely sentimental. Martin is neat, I am untidy. Martin is not social, I am good with people. Martin has never read a line of poetry in his life, I am a poet.

But in spite of, and often because of, those differences we fit very well. We are both independent. We share the same values in life. We are both easygoing and resilient. We make each other laugh. We love being parents. We have the same tastes in theatre and film, and while my range of reading matter is wider than Martin's we enjoy the overlap – part of my job in the family is sourcing Martin's reading material, just as it was on that first day we met.

As the year ticks down to that June morning in 2009, Martin, who has been working part-time for a few years, is making plans to retire. With his new dance passion, his goal in life is to notate and learn all 3,000 current folk dances. Work gets in the way.

With Martin retired, I will be left as the only breadwinner. Martin and I have always both worked, and for me the juggling trick, now that Amantha has grown up, is between work and writing.

For a few years now I have been unable to keep both balls in the air. The ongoing post-chemo fatigue, neck and back problems and the need to earn a living have meant that writing has been taking a distant back seat. The only way I am going to be able to write is to cut down on my patient hours. But with mine as the only income, that cut means I will also have to cut down on two of the things that bring me joy – books and craft materials. It has taken me a long time, but I have finally bitten the bullet and come to a decision. This June, I will cut down on some of my patient hours and give myself more time to write. Having made the decision, I am excited about it – the thought of having more free time and energy to write is exhilarating. This year, 2009, is going to be my year. June is my lodestone.

And then June comes.

15 July 2009

My brand of chickenpox seems to be exceptionally robust. I have been waiting for my pustules to turn black for what seems an eternity. While housebound this morning, I entertain myself by attempting to solve the mystery of the missing Visa card. It is now five weeks since I was told the replacement Visa card was on its way.

Today's investigations have involved several convoluted conversations with Sydney on the subject. I am now told that the Visa card was posted several days ago and should be at the local Elsternwick branch. A conversation with the Elsternwick branch is suggested. One lengthy conversation with the Elsternwick branch later and I am told there is no record of the card. They have had no notification that it was ever posted and they have certainly never received it.

Several further phone calls later and the Sydney office is crossing its heart and swearing that the new Visa card was indeed posted express on 3 July, several days ago.

'But it didn't get to me', I say. The NAB man, in the hurt tones of the unjustly accused, gives me the number of the Express Post envelope in which it was posted. I set about ringing the post office to track its trail.

'Yes', the post office finally says, 'it was posted on 3 July and arrived at its destination on the 8 July'.

'Its destination?' I repeat. 'Yes', she says. 'Cairns'.

'But I live in Caulfield', I squeak.

'Well it was sent to Cairns', she says.

'Cairns?' says the man at the local NAB branch. 'Why did they send it to Cairns?'

'You're the one who's supposed to tell me that', I say.

'Cairns', he repeats thoughtfully. His voice has the beginnings of an 'aha' note in it.

I can hear his thought processes. Cairns, Caulfield... They both start with 'C', don't they? Doesn't that mean they are the same thing?

When I ring the next morning he still has not heard from the person who was trying to track the card down somewhere in Cairns.

Meanwhile, of course, I still don't have a Visa card, and all the things that were automatically paid through it are beginning to run out. As they were automatic and invisible to me, I am met with a new surprise each day. The paper has not come. It was paid with the Visa. The milk and eggs have not come. They were paid with the Visa.

The Visa malfunction gets added to the phone malfunction, the computer malfunction and the chicken-pox malfunction. At some point, I reassure myself, the normal curve is bound to reassert itself in terms of the statistical probability of all these things going wrong in such a short space of time.

16 July 2009

Martin is continuing to become more and more dexterous with words. With his recovering ability to communicate comes the ability to tell me for the first time the full story of what happened in Frankston on the night he was admitted – when his symptoms turned from mild to devastating.

It is extraordinary to hear the story that has been unknown until now. As Martin tells me, I find myself being simultaneously thrilled that he can talk well enough to tell me and horrified at what I am hearing.

The only noticeable sign of a stroke when Martin was first admitted was a slowness in speech. He could still speak but simply had a bit of difficulty in finding and expressing his words. He could write normally and there was no paralysis in his arm or leg.

The CT scan didn't show up any bleeding, and the clot causing his symptoms was so small it didn't show up on the scan. He looked set to stay overnight and go home the next morning functioning fairly well and on the way back to normal.

Everything stayed like that overnight – no deterioration and minimal damage. Then at 5.30 in the morning Martin got up to use the toilet. He had eaten dinner at the hospital the evening before and was a touch constipated, so he was straining to get his bowels moving. And that was what did it. The straining on the toilet increased the blood pressure in his brain. That increase in pressure stressed the already fragile blood vessels damaged by the mini-stroke. The blood vessels burst under the strain, causing a massive bleed into Martin's brain.

As the blood vessels burst, Martin felt a sudden, odd sensation in his head. He became dizzy. When he went to lift his arm, he couldn't move it – the right side of his body was paralysed. He didn't understand what was happening. Somehow he stumbled his way back to bed but couldn't work out how to get the attention of a nurse – the function of a call button had become completely foreign to him. He lay there unable to communicate in any way until he was discovered by a nurse doing the rounds at 8.00 am. The genesis of that sudden terrible deterioration had remained unknown because in the weeks following, Martin could not speak to tell anyone.

It is shocking to hear this story. I had known somewhere in the back of my mind that straining on the toilet could temporarily raise blood pressure in the brain but it was filed under distant trivia never to be thought about. Spurred on by this information I do some investigation and discover an article in the reputable medical journal *Stroke* by researchers in the Netherlands (one of those oddly apt conjunctions of research topic and country of origin). They connect straining on the toilet with the bursting of aneurysms (malformed and fragile blood vessels) in the brain. 'We think it is feasible to advise persons with [brain aneurysms] to refrain from coffee drinking and to use laxatives when constipated', noted the researchers.

The damaged blood vessels surrounding a clot in the brain would have the same vulnerability as the blood vessels of an aneurysm, and I think to myself how easy it would have been to have given Martin a laxative or at least warn him, and similar patients, not to strain on the toilet. It is impossible to know, of course, whether Martin's blood vessels would have burst under some other strain in the days following his stroke, but at least this would have minimised one risk factor in those delicate post-stroke days.

The information about straining on the toilet goes into the folder in my mind labelled 'What I Know Now'. It is a folder that is becoming more and more voluminous. And it consists entirely of things that are not currently implemented by hospitals and yet are research-based and likely to improve the outcomes of stroke patients. This is not because our hospitals or medicos are below standard. It is simply due to the fact that hospitals are overcrowded, doctors and health therapists are overworked and time-poor, and research takes time, often a long time, to trickle down to the point where it is routinely implemented.

And the heavy workloads of medical and nursing staff have an impact in other areas of patient care as well. These range from the simple tasks of fetching a drink for a thirsty patient to the more complex and crucial aspects of care, such as interspecialist communication, the double-checking of medications and so on. When I say that I cannot imagine how one fares without someone to act as a patient-advocate, every doctor and nurse I have spoken to nods their head in violent agreement.

17 July 2009

I discover I have found the key to reversing the power balance between hospital visitors and staff. Get chickenpox, recover and visit the hospital. With my newly dried-up pustules, I arrive to visit Martin in hospital for the first time in two weeks. The nurses and doctors react with terror when they see me coming. As one, they shrink back against the walls squeaking piteously, 'Are you safe?'

And it is so good to be 'safe' again. Earlier this morning I took myself out for a walk in the sunshine. After walking for about an hour, I even dropped in to the supermarket – the thrill was extreme. Driving to the hospital, though, later in the morning, I was almost cross-eyed with fatigue. I kept wondering whether the windscreen was blurry or was it just me. It was me. Martin, in contrast, is as bright as the proverbial button. It is astonishing to see how much more he is able to do than when I saw him last, a fortnight ago. I am getting the sporadic visitor's-eye view of his progress as opposed to the day-to-day one I am used to and it is mind-blowing.

We go for a walk in the hospital grounds and he tells me the OTs are so pleased with him they will forgo the usual house-check before his homecoming in a little over a week. This comes as welcome news – ever since outwitting the OT on the occasion of Martin's first weekend visit, I have lived in fear of retribution in the form of the words 'Clear this mess'.

I have brought Martin a selection of magazines to read – *Newsweek*, *Time* and the like. Reading is now part of his 'homework' – he is not up to books yet but magazines with short newsy pieces are perfect. And it is also the first time I have seen Martin's new bed – he has organised himself into the window bed in his three-bed ward. With the screening curtain up it is almost like a private room (except, of course, for the other two occupants' snoring at night).

It is six weeks since Martin's stroke and it is exhilarating to think he will soon be home and institution-free.

18 July 2009

The nurses are learning not to cower when they see me and my progress through the hospital is now marked by relatively few expressions of terror. And my newly non-contagious state has meant that I can take Martin home for the weekend.

I continue to be amazed by how much more Martin can do with his right hand now. When he came home last time, his right arm was in a sling – he couldn't move his fingers at all and had no power in his arm. Now he can pick up objects, shake hands and use both hands when folding a shirt.

Even though Martin is using his right hand in lots of ways he was unable to before, he still has a way to go with fine motor control. This morning, when he was trying to send an email using his right hand, he pressed the wrong keys about fifty per cent of the time. Similarly, now that he can pick things up, the next step involves working on placing them where he wants them to be.

We have a post-birthday celebration for Martin at Denise and Walter's, to make up for the birthday I couldn't spend with him, and play Articulation – the word game I picked up pre-chickenpox. It involves trying to guess a word from clues, and although it is timed and fast, Martin manages to get one of the words first out of the team.

It is a wonderful weekend. And as an extra bonus, the pustules are continuing to get blacker and drier. Although I still wake up itching and aching and am experiencing intense post-chickenpox fatigue, I am thrilling to the joys of being non-infectious. Adult chickenpox has had the effect of putting me in touch with being a child again, with the associated list of 'firsts' that are so exciting. This list includes my first shower, my first clean hair, my first face-to-face contact without several metres of separation, my first clothes that are not old nighties turned inside out – the dazzling list goes on.

Life is looking good. I am well. Martin is doing brilliantly. We are on the home stretch and cruising.

20 July 2009

I arrive at the hospital today to find that Martin has had a spike of temperature at around 11.00 am. The hospital dashed into action with a battery of tests – chest X-rays, blood tests, urine tests and a special blood culture at Prince Edward Hospital - but the temperature responded to Panadol and was back to normal by lunchtime. The results of the blood and urine tests have yet to come through but we both feel reassured that something as simple as Panadol brought his temperature down.

I ring the hospital several times between patients and Martin's temperature is staying normal. Jane the Pain, Martin's medical resident, has instructed him to stay in bed and not go to physio or speech therapy. Martin is a touch frustrated about this edict.

I speak to Martin a couple more times after I come home from my visit in the evening and his temperature continues to remain normal. It looks as if it is just a brief bout with a garden-variety bug – the salvo of tests ordered by the hospital seem to both of us to be a bit like Jewish-mother overkill.

21 July 2009

Martin's temperature has stayed normal all night and he sounds good in my pre-breakfast phone call. The X-rays, urine tests and blood tests have all come back clear and Jane has given him the okay to go back to his usual schedule.

I pick him up for an extended lunchbreak and we both have a wry chuckle about the red-alert response the hospital went into for a small spike of temperature. It contrasts starkly with the lapses in hygiene that are routine on the wards – orderlies picking up glasses of juice for patients with their hands covering the rims, staff neglecting handwashing, the cursory cleaning routines in bathrooms that leave more grime than they clear away, and so on. By the time we return from lunch, we are relaxed and laughing.

That pretty much stutters to a silence as we re-enter the ward. Jane gestures impatiently at us.

'Where have you been?' she asks curtly. And before we can answer, she continues, 'Martin has to go straight onto antibiotics. Prince Edward says his blood culture is growing a nasty bacterium'.

Martin and I both struggle for our voices.

I recover mine first. 'What —' but Jane is on a roll.

'It's got to be given intravenously', she says, ignoring me, 'so he'll have to have a cannula inserted'.

And a nurse leads Martin off to attach a drip.

'What's the antibiotic?' I say.

'It's an antibiotic', Jane answers helpfully.

I try a different angle. 'Are there any side effects I need to know about?'

'No', says Jane. 'No side effects you need to know about'. And with that, dashes away before I can grab my wits, or her, for a second round of interrogation.

I try to hunt up a nurse. Martin has had the cannula inserted and has been ordered back to bed. Nurses, though, are in short supply. Even more so than usual, as this is the week of a big national rehab conference and all the consultants are at it and not here. Every ward is short-staffed.

Finally I catch a passing nurse. 'I want to know what antibiotic Martin has been put on'.

She gestures frantically. 'I'll check when I've finished dealing with Mr C'. And she disappears.

More time goes by. Nurses pass only infrequently, and every one I catch has to attend to something else before they can attend to me. Finally, time and logistics come in to bat for me. Martin's antibiotic infusion needs refilling. No nurse has yet deigned to talk to me but I follow them to the nurses' station and eavesdrop while they discuss Martin's antibiotic refill. To my horror, I catch the word vancomycin. It is one of the big guns of the antibiotic world. What on earth is the bug that has been found in Martin's blood?

Enquiries to the nurses about the nature of the bug meet with failure. Apparently, the Prince Edward report is in the computer and the computer can only be accessed by doctors. So where are the doctors? This question is met with shrugs. I try paging, searching and questioning anyone in a hospital outfit but Jane is nowhere to be found. By the time evening comes, it is clear I am not going to get any answers today.

22 July 2009

I arrive at South-Central this morning to discover that Martin has developed a sore foot and leg overnight. I finally manage to collar Jane, who looks at them and authoritatively pronounces the pain and inflammation to be result of the infection. Indeed, perhaps the fountainhead of the infection.

'If the inflammation goes down, we'll know the antibiotics are working', she says. And disappears before I have a chance to ask her what kind of infection it is.

It takes several more hours before I find her again by tracking the source of a chance aural snatch of her voice. She is tucked inside an alcove, going through medications with a nurse.

'What kind of bacterial infection does Martin have?' I say before she has time to get away.

'Mumble-mumble', she responds.

I track it phonetically, making a note to look it up on Dr Google.

'Is it a hospital infection?'

'No', she says, and looks interested for the first time. 'It's not usually found in the bloodstream. We can't understand how it got there'.

'Is it dangerous?'

'It's all under control', she says, the 'Whatever...' thought bubble reappearing over her head. 'The vancomycin is dealing with it'.

And then a pause. 'And Prince Edward is running tests to see if it's vancomycin-resistant'. And with that she has done her disappearing act again.

I am left with the question 'And if it *is* vancomycin-resistant?' hanging in the space she occupied mere milliseconds ago.

No one, of course, can tell me when the Prince Edward's conclusions re drug resistance are going to arrive, so Martin's foot becomes the source of all wisdom. According to Jane, if it gets better, the vancomycin is working. If it doesn't, the vancomycin is not.

It is not getting better. By the time I leave the hospital at night, Martin is unable to put any weight on it at all. He is also feeling miserable. The IV infusion has to be refilled every few hours. Half the time when the nurses top it up, the cannula is dislodged from the vein so that the vancomycin leaks into the surrounding tissue and causes him pain. The cannula then has to be reinserted, causing him even more pain. The nurses say this is a common occurrence and that Martin's body is 'rejecting the cannula'. I don't know if this is true or whether competence at cannula-insertion also counts…

23 July 2009

When I come in this morning, the infection is looking more localised in Martin's foot. I drag Jane over to have a look.

She gives it a cursory prod and says casually 'Yes, it's a septic shower caused by the bug'.

'A septic shower?'

She nods. 'It's a concentration of the bug that's in Martin's bloodstream'.

'But —'

She has already disappeared.

Since this began, Martin has been ordered to stay in bed and skip his therapies. In the absence of speech therapy, I have been buying up simple crossword and other word puzzles and going through them with Martin. He is restless and understandably impatient. Four days have ticked by without speech therapy and physiotherapy while he waits out this bug. I have still not been able to find out the results of the Prince Edward's investigations. Every last consultant seems to have been swept off to conference-land in an imitation of the Rapture at world's end. No one can tell me what is going on. All we can do is watch Martin's foot, which continues to be inflamed, tender and presumably septically showered.

Martin is irritated at being ordered to skip his speech and physio till he is better. I am antsy because Martin now has a bug that shouldn't be there floating around in his bloodstream, a bug that may or may not be being treated successfully by an antibiotic that is a king-hitter but may or may not be the right one.

I have discovered the name of the bug – *Enterococcus faecalis* – and from what I have read, once that particular bug gets into the bloodstream it becomes exceptionally nasty and is lethal unless successfully treated. Despite this, Martin is yet to see a consultant. Jane, who is very junior in the chain and whose middle name is

Incompetence, is the only medico who has come near him. I am getting distinctly worried.

I take to lurking around the nurses' station, picking up snatches of conversation. It seems to provide more information than the usual route of asking sensible questions. Late in the afternoon I hit paydirt. I hear one of the nurses casually mention that Dr C., a rehab consultant to one of the other wards, is going to be in the hospital at 11.00 am tomorrow.

24 July 2009

I arrive to be met with the news that the Prince Edward has rung to say vancomycin is indeed the right drug for Martin's bug. But Martin's foot is not getting better. What does that mean? The bug is not vancomycin-resistant but nevertheless is not getting knocked out by it. Nothing about this sounds good.

I go to the nurses' station. 'Martin needs to see a consultant', I say, doing my best to channel Arnold Schwarzenegger.

The nurses are unimpressed. 'The consultants are all at a conference', one says, barely bothering to look at me.

'Dr C. isn't', I counter assertively. 'I know he's going to be in the hospital this morning. Martin has to be seen by him'.

This time the nurse looks up, impressed by my handle on Secret Hospital Knowledge.

'I don't know what he's doing', she says.

'Well, get a message to him. Martin isn't getting better and he needs to be seen. I'll expect Dr C. to see him this morning'.

The nurse grudgingly nods.

And to our amazed relief, at 11.00 am promptly, a large man ambles into Martin's room. He is not carrying a tray, he is not limping, he is not stroke-damaged and he doesn't look like a nurse. Dr C. has arrived – a real-life, postgraduate-trained consultant in rehabilitation medicine. And he is staying in the same spot for more than one second.

I explain the scenario and what has been happening so far, ending up with Jane's septic shower theory.

I notice Dr C.'s eyebrows raise themselves slightly at this last point.

'Let's have a look', he says and proceeds to gently prod Martin's inflamed, tender foot.

'Nope', he says. 'It's not an infection'.

He muses to himself. 'It doesn't seem painful enough for gout. Might be fasciitis, caused by a strain on the foot. An anti-inflammatory ought to help'.

The pain in Martin's foot has also had a companion pain in Martin's calf since it began. Dr C. inspects it, thinks it is likely to be caused by muscle strain but orders an immediate scan to make sure it is not a blood clot given Martin's recent history.

I gasp slightly at this, with the recognition that I have not even thought of the blood clot possibility. And I should have. I know perfectly well that pain in a calf can indicate a blood clot with the potential to break free and cause damage to the heart, lungs or brain. I have been so focused on the septic shower theory that my vision has become tunnel.

Dr C. prescribes an anti-inflammatory, tells the nurses to organise a scan for this morning and breezes out, leaving us limp with relief at actually having seen someone competent for the first time this week.

A couple of hours after starting the anti-inflammatory meds, Martin is already noticing that his foot feels better. He is due for his scan in an hour and I head off to scout for more crosswords and puzzles to tide us over the coming weekend.

I arrive back home, breezy with relief that the 'septic shower' we have been agonising about for the last few days has been swept away with anti-inflammatories. I have been out scouring newsagents, bookstores and toyshops and have triumphantly managed to score a few new and appropriate word puzzles. And I have groceries and fruit for Martin's weekend at home tomorrow.

Bent over the fruit and vegetable stands in the supermarket, I had a sudden flashback to my dream of the night before. It was short but vivid. In it, I went to my kitchen cupboard at home to get some vegetables. Instead, I found two bananas on the shelf where potatoes, onions and the like normally live. For some reason I was happy to see the bananas and picked them up – I was particularly fascinated by the banana peel and gazed at it intently. The peel seemed important somehow, the word 'peel' imprinting itself in my mind. And there the dream ended.

I muse over this as I pick out non-banana produce. No meaning springs to mind. I toy with the image of the banana peel I was left with at the end of the dream. The last few weeks have certainly been skiddy, but I shy away from the other half of that famous saying that involves one foot on a banana skin. Anyway, I tell myself, the bananas had their skins on and there was something good about the peel – I was pleased to see it.

I arrive home ready to head out to South-Central and surprise Martin with a slice of his favourite apple pie for afternoon tea. Just before leaving the house, I phone South-Central to make sure he is back from his scan. Martin is not in his room, so I dial the nurses' station. The conversation runs as follows.

'It's Doris', I say brightly. 'Just checking to see if Martin's back from his scan'.

'Oh, yes', the nurse says. 'He's just coming back now'.

'Great', I say.

'But the ambulance is arriving at three', she continues.

'The what?'

'The ambulance', she repeats, with the patience of someone talking to a non-English-speaker. He's being transferred to the Prince Edward'.

'He's what?'

'He's being urgently transferred to the Prince Edward'.

'Why…? What…? No one's told me', I squawk. 'What's happening? Why is he going to the Prince Edward?' My voice is rising by the second.

'Oh, didn't they tell you? I'll find a nurse'.

'You *are* a nurse. Tell me why he's being transferred to the Prince Edward'.

'I'll have to get another nurse'.

Other nurse gets on the phone. 'I can't tell you why he's being transferred to the Prince Edward. You'll have to talk to a doctor'.

'Well, get me a doctor on the phone'.

Another nurse gets on the phone.

'I can't tell you anything, you need to talk to his doctor'.

'Well, tell Jane I need to talk to her', I shriek.

'Oh, Jane's busy'.

'Tell Jane to ring me immediately'.

Two hours later, Jane rings.

'The bug is too serious for us to treat at South-Central', she says. 'The Prince Edward Infectious Diseases Department insisted we transfer Martin immediately because we don't have the facilities to take care of him. And they are changing his medication. He's going to be on IV benzylpenicillin for two weeks'.

'Why? What changed since this morning?'

'A new result came through and they said the bug was too serious for us to deal with. And it's most sensitive to penicillin. He's being transferred urgently to the Prince Edward'.

And she hangs up.

Martin is already on his way in the ambulance and no one can give me any more information. I phone Amantha and in a mutual state of escalating tension we weave our way through peak-hour traffic to the Prince Edward.

It takes a while for the hospital staff to locate Martin but they finally find him in a temporary bed. Amantha and I get there to find a doctor in the middle of examining him.

'Hi', she says to us. 'I'm Kathy. I'm a registrar in the Infectious Diseases Unit. Martin's been transferred to our care'.

She finishes the physical examination calmly and competently, then gives us a full and clear explanation of what has happened, the first one we have received since this began.

The blood culture run by the Prince Edward has picked up a bug that is normally found in the bowel, where it does no particular harm. If it gets into the bloodstream, however, it becomes deadly, as this particular bug has a predilection for heading for the heart and setting up shop there. Once ensconced in the heart it becomes like one of those nasty tenants who don't make any noise or create noticeable external disturbance for most of their tenancy but leave the place wrecked when they exit. If the bug remains undetected once it has settled in the heart, it will kill.

Although the echocardiograms Martin has had so far have not shown up any cardiac damage, he will have to have a more thorough form of echocardiogram referred to by its acronym of TOE. The TOE in fact operates from the opposite end to the appendages of the feet. It stands for transoesophageal echocardiogram and involves inserting a probe through the oesophagus to produce a much clearer picture of what is happening in the heart. It necessitates an anaesthetic and sedation, and Kathy will put Martin on the list for it.

In the meantime, she will organise a bed for Martin in the Infectious Diseases Unit. Apologetically, she explains to us that while the beds in the IDU are normally single-bed wards, because of this winter's flu epidemic, the single beds are taken so Martin may have to share a two-bed ward. Clearly, she has not visited South-Central lately or she might not be sounding so apologetic.

She shakes our hands and prepares to leave. I shake hands particularly heartily – it is so refreshing to actually have a doctor who a) is not Jane, b) knows what she is doing, and c) is prepared to take the time to explain it. Just as she is about to exit, I realise it would be good to know her surname in case I need to contact her. I glance at her Prince Edward identification badge and there it is: Dr Kathy Peel. And, just as in my dream, this is indeed a peel I am glad to see.

Later in the evening I ring Martin. The expected transfer to the luxury of the Infectious Disease Unit has not happened; the flu is doing too good a job of infecting Melbourne's populace. Instead, Martin has been shifted to the old, old part of the Prince Edward and is housed in a tiny, grotty two-bed ward in the Neurology Department. He is sounding pretty miserable.

Update, 25 July 2009

This morning I left the house bright and early but failed to arrive at the Prince Edward bright and early due to traffic. Tomorrow I will clearly have to change my plans to less bright and more early. It took about an hour of circumnavigating the rambling hospital to find the Neurology Ward. No signs are necessary to let you know you have arrived. The soundtrack does the trick. The first thing I heard was someone screaming over and over – 'Help, they're holding me prisoner. Somebody help me!' At first I looked around instinctively for help. But the nurses were moving past without taking the slightest notice and the voice was taking on the quality of a stuck record. This had to be the place.

Martin's ward was indescribably tiny. There is barely room for his bed, let alone his belongings. His ward-mate was entertaining a string of visitors who were braying loudly and practically sitting on top of Martin. And in addition, the ancient bathroom, which Martin investigated this morning, is half-broken and distinctly grubby – as well as its standard accumulative grime, his roommate urinates very haphazardly.

The bathroom doesn't even boast a shelf on which to rest various essential implements, which means that in order to brush his teeth, Martin has to trek constantly back and forth between his room and the bathroom: from the bathroom to his room to fetch the toothbrush and toothpaste, back to his room to return the toothpaste and keep the toothbrush, back to the bathroom to brush his teeth, then back to his room to put the toothbrush down and fetch the glass, back to the bathroom with the glass to rinse his mouth, and so on. This constant zigzagging makes the whole process a hundred times more arduous and energy-consuming than it should be.

On top of that, the benzylpenicillin IV needs to be changed every four hours. And that means every four hours day and night. Add to this the very loud snoring of his bedside neighbour and Martin has not even had the chance to catch anything remotely resembling sleep.

I made a note to bring Martin a plastic toiletries bag with a strap that he can sling over his shoulder to alleviate the need for zigzagging backwards and forwards between bathroom and ward. I have a small collection of these toiletry bags, which have been waiting patiently for their chance to go on a *holiday. Doubtless, this one will get a shock as it discovers that the Riviera resort for which it believes it is intended has turned into the ancient grunge of a decaying hospital bathroom.*

The benzylpenicillin schedule and neighbour are less easily solved.

At mid-morning, we set out to investigate the delights of the Prince Edward cafeteria. I used to work at the Prince Edward fifteen years ago. Back then my chief source of entertainment was the hot chocolate machine. Now there is an array of shiny shops as well as a couple of cafeterias. We sat at a table with tea and cake and felt remarkably like civilians, as opposed to army combatants. It was a refreshing change, and we were savouring it when suddenly the loudspeaker blared out Martin's name and instructed him to report to 5 West immediately. We jumped guiltily and scrambled for the lifts, expecting to be court-martialled on arrival.

Instead, we found Kathy doing her rounds with a resident in tow. She explained that she was trying to get the TOE scheduled as soon as possible but that it is hard to get a definite time confirmed. The Radiology Department operates on a rather whimsical schedule for inpatients who are not deemed emergency-level urgent. Essentially, we will know that Martin has an appointment for his TOE when they come to get him. She is also organising some other body scans to see if the bug has taken up a wider residence in Martin's body.

Kathy said that if it turns out that Martin's heart is fine and the bug is in decline or gone, then it will most likely be a seven-day IV course of benzylpenicillin and Martin can go home. If, however, the TOE shows evidence of the bug in Martin's heart, then it will necessitate a six-week course of IV antibiotic and Martin will have to stay in hospital.

In the meantime, Martin's rehabilitation program has been prematurely broken off and the Prince Edward shows no signs of producing any substitutes. So I got out my sack of word games and we set to work. Our word-guessing games were regularly enlivened by Martin's roommate getting in and out of bed. As he was wearing a hospital gown that was not done up in the back, we were getting even more of the mooning flashes than those a secured hospital gown provides. All in all it is proving to be disturbingly reminiscent of the good old days with Trevor. Martin, in fact, is feeling downright sentimental about the old South-Central ward and I am reminded of the rubber stamp I purchased that simply and profoundly states 'Nothing bad is good until something worse happens'.

26 July 2009

Today Radiology comes to the party and Martin is given notice that his TOE is scheduled for tomorrow. Apparently, the only reason we are being given the luxury of notice is because Martin has to fast before the procedure, as it requires a general anaesthetic. We are told it will happen first thing tomorrow morning.

On the assigned morning, I have calculated that because of the anaesthetic, Martin will be out to the world for a couple of hours. I am using this time to try to find fiddly little children's puzzles that require fine motor skills. Of course, the skills mustn't be too fine, but neither must they be too easy. As Martin's self-appointed combination physio and OT in lieu of the real thing, I am scouting shops for the appropriate toys. Having found several – peg puzzles, pattern-making games and assorted others – I head back to the Prince Edward expecting to find a just-waking Martin.

To my surprise, he is alert and awake, chugging down morning tea in his room and attacking a couple of scones. He tells me the doctors – Kathy, the radiologist and another unfamiliar medico came in to tell him afterwards that they had seen a small patch of infection in his heart. This means he has officially been diagnosed with endocarditis. He is fuzzy on the details and cannot remember much of what they said. This is entirely understandable, given he had only barely emerged from a general anaesthetic at the time. I set out to find his doctors to hear the full extent of what sounds like the bad news we had been hoping to avoid.

Finally, I locate Kathy and ask her what the radiologist saw on Martin's heart. I am about to discover, however, that the rules of Looking-Glass Land have come into effect at the Prince Edward.

Kathy tells me she cannot tell me what the radiologist saw until the radiologist's formal report has come in.

'When will that be?' I ask.

The response is a shrug. The timing of radiologists' reports seems to be in sync with the roll-the-dice-and-take-a-punt timing of radiological scans. A few days seems the most likely bet.

'A few days' rolls off the tongue lightly as a mere snippet of time. Not so when you are waiting to hear news that will classify you as either on the way to recovery or very significantly sicker than you thought you were.

'But you told Martin what you saw on the TOE'.

'But he's the patient'.

'He was groggy with anaesthetic and doesn't remember what you told him'.

'We can only tell the patient'.

'But I'm the patient's nearest relative. I have the medical power of attorney. After any surgery the surgeon comes out and talks to the relatives, not the patient'.

Kathy shakes her head. She is sorry but she cannot do it. Apparently policy dictates that the news is allowed to be given to the semi-conscious patient but not the fully conscious spouse.

Kathy does tell me, however, that tomorrow Martin will be having a PICC line inserted. PICC stands for peripherally inserted central catheter. It is a long, thin, flexible tube inserted into a peripheral vein, typically through a vein in the upper arm, and extended so that the tip terminates in a large vein in the chest near the heart. This allows intravenous access to any drugs running through the PICC line. It means that at least Martin will not have to go through the painful process of having the cannula replaced every forty-eight hours.

27 July 2009

While we wait the required number of days for the radiologist's report, life on the Neurology Ward settles down to the new normal. I take Martin on regular walks around the hospital for exercise. Each time we re-enter the ward, it is made clear that this is indeed the Neurology Ward. The patient who believes he has been kidnapped and held against his will still believes that and regularly calls for anyone passing to aid in his escape. Various other colourful calls and choruses trill through the air. The assorted delusions and hallucinations being experienced and commented upon by the occupants of 5 West would easily populate a library of books in the magic realism style.

Martin's roommate, who has turned out to be such a genial fellow that his poor aim and sartorial inclinations have been forgiven, tells me of an unexpected visitor who arrived while Martin and I were on a walk.

A tiny elderly lady wandered into the room. Martin's roommate opened his eyes, sleepy from a nap and enquired in a gentlemanly fashion whether she was lost.

'No', she announced firmly.

Was there anything he could help her with? Was there anything she needed?

'Yes', she pronounced equally firmly, leaping into bed with him. 'I know exactly what I need'.

His efforts to free himself took on the panicked aspects of someone attempting to extricate himself from the embrace of a capuchin monkey clinging on for dear life. Eventually, a nurse wandered in to help with the extraction.

28 July 2009

The radiologist's report arrives back faster than expected. As conveyed by Kathy, it is the classic combination of good news/bad news. The bad news is there is a small area of infection in the heart, which means Martin will have to have six weeks of IV antibiotic. The good news is that the area is small rather than large. At some point, she says, we will have to organise a consultation with Cardiology to see what they have to say about the extent of damage and whether it will require surgery. Kathy also adds that 'something' was also seen in Martin's spleen, indicating that the bug had done the grand around-the-world tour of Martin's body. Hopefully, any nests of infection will be killed by the heavy doses of antibiotics running through Martin's veins.

As I mentally steel myself for the possibility of this new, unexpected surgery, Kathy moves on to what is now a regular theme in doctors' consults on Martin – the big questions of 'why' and 'how'. A new mystery has opened up. How did this bug, which is not normally found in the bloodstream, get there? Why did it arrive during Martin's stay at South-Central? It is not a standard hospital infection, so the usual explanations about bugs during hospital stays don't apply. Kathy professes herself mystified, as do the rest of the IDU consultants with whom she has spoken.

29 July 2009

Last night, I had an odd dream. When I wake this morning, all I can remember from the dream is a vivid scene that seemingly make no sense. There is an image of a sewing machine with the back end warped, driven into an odd angle from pressure. It is particularly strange because I keep thinking in the dream that it should have been the front end that was damaged, not the back – as if the damage was the wrong way around. In the dream, I called Martin in to show him – I simply couldn't understand how the back end was damaged rather than the front end – it felt wrong. Martin seemed to think it was fixable but as he was fixing it, a clear thin piece of transparent plastic, shaped like a razor dropped from the machine and half-embedded itself into his arm. I knew a doctor had to take it out so that it didn't break off. And that is all I can remember when I wake.

I have no idea what those images mean, but I wake with the sense that the dream is trying to tell me something about Martin's symptoms, that somehow his various illnesses and the mysteries around them are connected to the two images in the dream – the damage on the sewing machine, which is the wrong way around, and the plastic razor.

As I multi-task early this morning, rushing around getting ready for a day of hospital with Martin and then patients in the late afternoon, I am also thinking about what on earth my two dream images mean.

The sewing machine image is obviously important. I was focused in the dream on the fact that the damage was the wrong way around – it should have been at the front not the back of the machine. It makes me think of Elias Howe, who invented the sewing machine and how he nearly gave up because he kept trying to construct it with the needle the wrong way up.

The other focus of the dream was the transparent razor, which reminds me of Occam's razor. When the term Occam's razor is used within the medical context, it refers to a single diagnosis that covers all the observed symptoms.

As I let the above two snippets float around in my mind, I begin to think that maybe the two things the dream was saying are 1) you are looking at things from the wrong end, and 2) there is a single explanation for all the symptoms.

And then it occurs to me that after Martin's benign prostate operation back in late February, he had an unexplained fever for a day that was treated with Panadol and antibiotics, but no blood test or culture was recommended or carried out. What if the fever was actually signalling the arrival of the bug? It could have entered Martin's body via the surgical procedure on his prostate. Perhaps the fever and outward symptoms were cleared by the antibiotic but the bug had already headed for Martin's heart, made a nest for itself and stayed relatively unnoticed, as can happen with this bug, until a bit of the bug colony broke off and headed for the brain, where it caused the stroke.

In other words, according to this explanation, the infection came first rather than last, lay low for a while, caused the stroke and then, weeks later, reared its head again in the bloodstream with fever at South-Central and this time was investigated and discovered. Voilà, Occam's razor.

When I arrive at the Prince Edward, I discover that Martin, too, has been doing some thinking and is also wondering what that post-prostate fever signified. I corner Kathy and ask her if this is a possible explanation and she says it is certainly possible. Then just as I arrive home to see patients, Martin rings to say that the cardiologist had arrived with the final report. When Martin told him the theory about the February post-prostate infection, the cardiologist said that made absolute sense and he was sure that was the correct explanation. Mysteries solved.

The cardiologist had also looked through the radiologist's reports and films, and reported the good news that the infection was very small and wouldn't need any surgical intervention. A sigh of relief is breathed by all.

What is startling to think about now is that in this new context, Martin's stroke was literally, and bizarrely, a stroke of luck. If Martin hadn't had the stroke, no one would have been investigating his heart. And furthermore, he wouldn't have been in South-Central when he ran that temperature for a day. If it had happened at home, Panadol would have brought the temperature down and there would have been no South-Central Rehab to act as 'Jewish mother' and go into overdrive with blood investigations. If these events had not occurred, the endocarditis would not have been discovered and the infection would have continued to grow until it proved fatal. Because of the stroke, Martin's endocarditis has been discovered in time to save his life.

30 July 2009

Martin has had his PICC line inserted and is very pleased with it. He is enjoying being cannula-free and particularly enjoying the absence of painful intrusions into veins as nurses attempt to reinsert stray cannulas. Less enjoyable, however, is the news that his neighbour is being discharged today.

Having sampled a fair distribution of the Neurology Ward's occupants from their contribution to the ongoing corridor chorus, we are somewhat apprehensive as to who Martin's new ward-mate will be.

Much to our surprise, and in keeping with modern co-ed institutional thinking, 'he' is a 'she', an elderly woman who is on major doses of haloperidol, an antipsychotic drug, so that she spends a fair amount of time semi-comatose. In her few waking moments, she vociferously proclaims the hospital is trying to poison her through her food. Depending on your culinary fancies, you may or may not agree with her.

My email updates over the last few days have been relatively short as I am so tired I can barely put two words together. Getting to the Prince Edward in time to get a parking spot of more than an hour's duration requires rising before the crack of dawn. As I stay in the hospital for most of the day, street parking several blocks away offers a less prohibitive expense than the hospital car park. It is miserable, however, in the grip of a very cold winter, to be continually trekking back and forth to feed parking meters.

When I am not at the hospital, I am either seeing patients or out on the constant search for more word games and puzzles requiring fine hand-motor control. Yesterday, I hit on the idea of knitting as an excellent way for Martin to exercise his hands and for a moment got quite excited at the thought of a small cottage industry in the person of Martin producing all the knitted garments I have ever coveted. Martin, however, is not quite so excited. His interest is only piqued when I show him a photo of a particularly intricate piece of ribbing. Unfortunately, it doesn't come with instructions.

He is due for a series of scans and tests in the next few days as the doctors want to leave no medical stone unturned. This morning he is having a CT of the colon and daily ECGs are on the cards. Another MRI of the brain is also planned. I had to remind the doctors there was actually an MRI taken four weeks ago in existence. The conversation went thus.

Prince Edward doctor: We want to organise an MRI for Martin.

Me: Martin had a brain MRI done four weeks ago.

Doctor: But this MRI we want to order is a special one, designed to look at the blood vessels of the brain.

Me: The one he had four weeks ago was looking for an AVM [arteriovenous malformation], so I imagine that would look at blood vessels.

Doctor: Did he really have that done four weeks ago? What hospital did it?'

Me: The Prince Edward.

Doctor: Huh? We never saw that.

31 July 2009

Today Martin's female roommate seems to be on a lowered dose of haloperidol. The effect is to make her more vocal and to give her greater clarity and precision with regard to the topic she is vocalising about. Apparently, it is not just the rather vague 'hospital' wanting to poison her, it is actually the boss of the hospital who wants to kill her. She has also spent the day conversing with herself (or some hallucinatory companion). She has a child-like, breathy voice, so the effect has a very Baby Jane (as in *Whatever Happened to...*) quality that is rather eerie. I am hoping she and her conversational companion will sleep soundly tonight. Waking up to that voice in the darkness would be deeply unnerving.

1 August 2009

Today there is some exciting news – a single room in the Infectious Diseases Unit has finally been found. And what a room! It is the equivalent of a 4-star hotel room. It is in a separate building, which is dedicated to the IDU. After the challenge of finding my way to a new location – about a block away from the main Prince Edward building, I am knocked out on viewing this mini-paradise. Martin's room is amazingly spacious and airy. There is a little balcony looking out onto a garden, a modern ensuite bathroom and, most excitingly for me, a recliner chair.

The drive home after hospital involves rapid stopping and starting at several shops to get objects such as a tray (for the jigsaw I bought for Martin yesterday), a colouring-in book with fine detail, for Martin to practice fine motor skills, and a cunning device at the toyshop that involves small beads that stick onto a frame in complicated patterns. Yesterday I bought Martin a very swish version of Boggle and printed out a pile of tongue twisters for him to practise, along with a few more word-puzzle books. This is all enough to keep Martin busier than the average Year 12 student.

2 August 2009

To keep us entertained today, Martin's PICC line has begun to leak. At the moment it is not leaking badly and the nurse is unsure why it is happening. The two possibilities are a) a faulty PICC line, or b) an infection. Obviously we are hoping for a) but while the PICC line is in situ, we have no way of knowing. The nurse is hoping the problem will clear up by itself. The doctor is due on rounds tomorrow.

By evening, the PICC line's leakage rate is rising. Although not quite up to the running-tap level, it is getting very close to a speed-walking one. The registrar on duty is called and announces it will have to be taken out and that Martin will be back on the hated cannulas until such time as someone who is expert at installing PICC lines is available. The tip of the PICC line will be sent off to Pathology to see if there is an infection. Martin is understandably feeling a bit down in response. Within another twenty-four hours, however, Martin will become the proud possessor of a new PICC line, this one inserted more expertly than its predecessor and watertight.

3 August 2009

The day is dragging on when suddenly Martin's consultant in the IDU arrives, presents himself in full view and remains stationary for more than five minutes. He introduces himself as Alex. I intuit his consultant status by watching the interplay of power/status/deference between Alex and Kathy, the IDU registrar. Alex turns out to be very good – on the ball, an excellent communicator, and he gives lots of time for questions and clear answers.

The CT of Martin's colon and spleen yesterday showed that the colon was fine but the spleen had something they were unsure about. After the regular meeting with the radiologists tomorrow, the IDU people will know more about that. Alex doesn't seem too worried about it and mentions as an aside that there was no sign of cancer. This gives us a slight turn, as we weren't aware they were looking for cancer. Alex also mentions that the most dangerous period when treating an infection of the heart, such as Martin's, is in the first forty-eight hours, as there is a chance that bits of the crusty infection will break off and cause strokes. We are both rather relieved to have passed the critical stage without knowing it, especially as the critical stage was being managed in South-Central Rehab under Jane the Pain.

Kathy also mentions the exciting possibility that Martin may be able to go home at some time under the auspices of the Prince Edward's 'Hospital In The Home' service. This wondrous service allows certain patients to return home, with daily visits from Prince Edward nurses to monitor their progress. As Martin still has some weeks of IV treatment to go, his ability to return home depends on the availability of a portable IV machine. Kathy tells us that as soon as one becomes available, she is happy for Martin to go home. The news of this possibility has us fizzing with excitement.

We return from a walk outside to the heady news that a portable IV pump will become available tomorrow and Martin will be going home. The nurse explains that we will be given a lesson in the mechanics of the machine and that a nurse will visit daily to check it and hand over the next twenty-four hours' worth of antibiotics to be fed through it.

4 August 2009

The morning is spent impatiently awaiting the doctors' visits, nurses' briefings, pharmacist's visit, all of which have to happen before we can pack the bags of stuff accumulated over two months in hospital into the car and head for home.

Martin is now attached to his new best buddy, the pump, twenty-four hours a day. The nurse came in earlier to hook Martin up to his portable pump and, some time afterwards, Martin, ever the engineer, realised there was a much more efficient way to trail the tube, which would enable him to put his jumper on without having to thread it through the pump first. The nurse is now planning to do it Martin's way for any future patients.

The device pumps the antibiotic mixture steadily into Martin's veins throughout the day and night. If it gets blocked, it will emit a piercing shriek. As will anyone else within 100 metres of it. Once a week we will journey in to the Infectious Diseases Outpatients Clinic and twice a week Martin will have speech, physio and OT sessions as an outpatient at South-Central. In between those visits he will be doing speech and physio homework so he, and I, are going to be kept busy. Martin will be on the IV pump for four to six more weeks and then on an oral antibiotic for months afterwards and perhaps for life.

There is a raft of papers to be signed before we can leave. Martin is so keen to sign that he practically grabs the papers from the nurse's hand. And then finally it is all done – we are free to leave. For the first time, after months as a hospital inpatient, Martin is coming home.

Part 2

5 August 2009

Martin is ecstatic to be home at last. It is two months, almost to the day, since the stroke. The difference in Martin is extraordinary. He can now have long conversations, although he still has the accent and slow, precise articulation of someone for whom English is a late-learned language, and his intonation doesn't sound like his old natural voice. What he most sounds like is a German-born man for whom English is a second language. Oddly enough, Martin was actually born in Munich, where his parents, who had survived the war hiding in a bunker constructed by his father, were searching for a way out of Europe. He was still a pre-verbal baby when he arrived in Australia, however, so German was never a native language.

He has also now graduated to cursive writing with his right hand, which means he is doing better than a lot of youngsters these days, for whom cursive script is predicted to be on the way to becoming a lost art due to the prevalence of keyboards. His writing is smaller than it used to be but his signature is recognisably the same. All his doctors are stunned by his progress and he is the pin-up boy at South-Central – their star patient whose story is told to give other patients hope.

And today Martin had a phone call on his mobile. It was from the NAB branch in Cairns who wanted to know why he hadn't come in to pick up his Visa card!

It is blissful having Martin home again. He is luxuriating in having his own bed, his own couch, his own bathroom, his own familiar home cooking, his own privacy and, of course, his own family. The list goes on and on. And the 'own' that precedes each of these nouns is not just there for emphasis or decoration. It speaks profoundly of the loss of self that accompanies being a patient, the loss of your own place in life, psychologically as well as spatially.

The personality changes that accompanied Martin's emergence from the stroke have been sustained. He has continued to be a 'softer' version of his old self – more caring and empathic, with a gentleness about him that touches me deeply. At least half a dozen times a day we exchange spontaneous 'I love you's' in a way we have not done for decades. It is like falling in love all over again. Martin can feel the changes in himself. He describes himself post-stroke as more emotional than his previous super-rational self. He is still logical and calm but feels emotions more easily and intensely than before. Because he is more in touch with his own emotions, he is now also more empathically in touch with those of others.

7 August 2009

The portable IV pump to which Martin is attached needs to be fed every twelve hours in a way rather similar to, but more complicated than, a carthorse's chaff bag. Martin's engineering mind has taken the process in its stride and he is managing the rather fiddly details expertly. A nurse arrives once a day to deliver new bags of antibiotics and check the drip. Once a week the nurse will change the dressing over the PICC line. Occasionally, Martin will need to change the battery. All fine and doable.

Complacency, of course, comes with its own warning label – get too used to things and you are asking for trouble. After a few pleasantly smooth days, today starts off with a morning visit by a very sloppy Prince Edward home nurse who has come to check the drip. She breezily assures us that a minor overnight leak that has developed in Martin's new antibiotic container is 'no problem'.

'Just keep it vertical', she says.

And we believe her.

It is a windy, rainy winter morning. Not a good day to walk outside. So to get some exercise, I bundle Martin off to an indoor mall. It is very long and not very crowded on a weekday – ideal for indoor walking.

We set off to circumnavigate the mall. I detour into a shop and Martin is happy to keep on walking. We each have mobile phones to keep in contact with each other and he is enjoying the freedom of walking on his own. After all, nothing can go wrong – the nurse said just to keep the drip vertical.

I have been in the shop for all of two minutes when my phone rings. It is Martin and he has retreated to the benches at the entrance of the mall and needs me to be there smartly. The drip has not understood the nurse's instructions. It has been kept vertical but it is very disobediently leaking like a fire hydrant.

When I turn the corner I find Martin sitting disconsolately surrounded by a spreading yellow puddle at his feet. Passing shoppers are keeping a wary distance. To my horror, I also notice a large air bubble poised halfway between the beginning of the feed-line and the vein offering entrance into Martin's circulatory system. No one has said anything about air bubbles and the drip. I know that if air bubbles get into the blood system they can be dangerous. Is this one of those instances? The bubble is slowly but definitely working its way upwards. Will it be transported into Martin's veins along with the antibiotic fluid? What will that mean?

Of course, both of us have left the house without the phone number for the Prince Edward At Home service. I ring South-Central Hospital, who put me through to the Prince Edward, who in turn put me through to Prince Edward At Home service.

By this time Martin is collecting puddles, plural, around him and we are watching the large bubble of air in the pump edge closer and closer to the spot where the tube enters his vein.

The Prince Edward nurse tells us to head for home, change the feedbag and make sure it stays vertical. By the time I get off the phone, however, the bubble has completed its journey upwards and has disappeared into the pump en route to Martin.

We get into the car and drive home in the pelting rain, wondering all the time what the bubble is doing. Halfway home, Martin's phone rings. It is Prince Edward At Home again. This time the nurse tells us we have to come straight in to the Prince Edward

Infectious Diseases Clinic. One of the head IDU consultants has decided to review Martin's case and thinks he needs a second antibiotic. He has to get to the Prince Edward urgently.

'But why?' I say.

'I can't tell you', says the nurse. 'You'll have to talk to the people at the clinic'.

And the phone goes dead before I can pose even the first of all the questions she cannot answer.

Martin and I exchange panicked glances. Why is the medication being changed at this late date – two weeks into the process? Does this mean the current medication is not working? Is the bug resisting treatment? Has something new and sinister shown up in the blood work?

So, with Martin dripping all over the car and our anxieties raised by what this new piece of news means, we manage to make it home, change the feedbag and pack an overnight bag in case this new turn of events means Martin is back in hospital again.

Once at the Prince Edward, we face a long and unnerving wait to be seen in the ID Clinic. Finally it is our turn and at last our questions can be answered.

It turns out the reviewing consultant has concluded that the bug that had taken up residence in Martin's heart was so dangerous it was best to king-hit it with two antibiotics rather than just the one. The new antibiotic is the one considered third best for this bug.

'Third best?' I query.

'Yes', the answer comes. 'Benzylpenicillin, the one that Martin is currently on, is the one considered second best'.

'But what about the one that's considered best for this bug?'

'Oh, that's the antibiotic that Martin's bug is resistant to'.

This is news to us. We had previously been told that benzylpenicillin was 'the best drug' for killing Martin's bug. Technically, of course, this is true, as the bug is resistant to number one on the list. We, however, had interpreted that statement to mean that Martin was being treated with the absolute, top-of-the-line, research-proven head-of-the-list killer of his bug. It is unnerving to realise he is having to make do with second best. And even more unnerving to realise that the consultant is so unsure of second-best's ability to take out this bug that he is adding third-best to the stable. It feels a little like putting all your money on a win on a horse race but being unable to bet on the horse most likely to win the race.

I also get the answer to my next question, about the air bubble that filled me with dread as I watched it seemingly disappear up the tube and into Martin's veins. The pump, it turns out, has an automatic filter for bubbles. We were, of course, left blissfully ignorant of this safety device.

As she attaches Martin to the new antibiotic, the nurse tells us that this addition will necessitate two home nurse visits a day instead of the one we were originally on and that Martin has to stay in the Prince Edward for a few hours to make sure he has no allergic reactions to it. Luckily, his body is happy to identify the new treatment as a friend and he is unplugged and released just in time for us to negotiate the Friday-afternoon peak-hour traffic on our route home.

14 August 2009

As the days have gone on we have been uniformly impressed by the quality of the Prince Edward At Home service. The slack nurse is the only instance we encounter of below-par care. And the freedom it gives us is invaluable.

Today we have our first Infectious Diseases outpatient appointment. We have come with the usual list of questions typed out. The most important one is how do we know if the medication has killed the bug?

In the past, we have been given varying answers to this. Averaged out, they amount to 'There's no way of knowing that it's been wiped out everywhere'.

This registrar says, in response to my question, that they were using a blood marker that measures inflammation (the CRP – C-reactive protein–marker) to monitor progress, and that the marker had been steadily going down and was in fact now at normal levels, which is very good news. The problem is that while this looks very promising, they cannot know for sure whether the bug is dead or just dormant. That is why Martin will be continuing on oral antibiotics for months after his six weeks of IV antibiotics are over. There is still controversy over how long patients should remain on the antibiotics, with many specialists maintaining that because of the risk of the infection re-emerging, patients should in fact be on antibiotics for life. Luckily, these are decisions we can put off till further down the track.

The good news for now is that the inflammation levels are down, there is no blood evidence of the bug and Martin's six weeks will be up on 1 September – very appropriately the first day of spring. And he will be carolling away and leaping, if not in the fields, at least around the wooden dance floor of a folk-dancing class, the instant he is freed of his metal and plastic companion.

I ask the registrar if the segment of bug colony that broke off from the heart valve and caused the stroke was a bit of live bug or dead bug. He says that is a good question and the answer, again, is they don't know. It is unnerving to think of such a deadly bug being alive in both Martin's brain and heart during all those weeks we were unaware of it.

After getting home from our Prince Edward appointment, Martin and I decide that an entertaining video is on the menu. It is a ten-minute walk to the video shop and the winter weather is in a kindly mood. We enjoy the stroll and the experience of browsing through the shelves of movies. The atmosphere is somewhat disturbed, though, by an irritating and incessant beeping sound, which I assume is coming from the shop's computer system.

'How do they stand working in a place with that constant noise?' I say to Martin.

I glance over to the young man at the counter but he seems unperturbed by the sound.

We choose our videos rather hurriedly and exit, eager to get away.

As we walk down the street I am amazed by the carrying power of the sound. Even though we are about fifty metres from the shop it is still clearly audible.

'That sound has incredible penetration', I remark.

Martin nods in agreement.

We walk faster. But the sound seems to be breaking all distance records – we can still hear it just as clearly as we could in the shop.

It takes another ten minutes before we realise it is not the sound that is carrying, it is we who are carrying the sound. It is coming from Martin's antibiotic feedbag, which has been insistently trying to tell us that it is hungry and wants more battery.

19 August 2009

Martin is only now beginning to recognise how extraordinary the speed and extent of his recovery from the stroke has been. His doctors are all uniformly amazed at how far he has come and the extent of his recovery from a position that carried with it a very gloomy prognosis. Although all his doctors at the time were pessimistic about his recovery, Martin had taken on board my continual reassurances that he would get better. He had always believed what I was saying and simply assumed he would make a good recovery.

While chatting to Martin some time after his return home, Cindy asks, 'Did you ever think you wouldn't get better?'

Martin shakes his head emphatically. 'Doris always told me about the new research and the ways my brain could repair itself, so I always thought I'd do it'.

Afterwards, Cindy says to me, 'Isn't it wonderful that he always thought he would get there. You and I, with too much knowledge, would have felt much more pessimistic and depressed about our odds'.

And it is true.

Part of what Martin is now working on in his speech therapy sessions is getting back his normal voice and intonation. His speech therapist is getting him to say the same sentence several times, using a variety of emotional tones (angry, happy, pleading, and so on). This is working well – Martin's voice and accent are markedly more melodic as he does this. And of course it appeals to the thespian in him – Martin is an excellent natural actor.

I have also unearthed two copies of sketches from British comedy duo Morecambe and Wise for Martin and me to read out loud Hopefully they will provide a few laughs as well as speech practice. In addition, I am on the lookout for the lyrics of enjoyable songs, as singing will also help Martin's voice return to its normal melodic intonations. I am anticipating a ten-minute singing session daily. Given the quality of my singing, this may force Martin into a faster recovery than planned in an effort to avoid the torture.

All has been going smoothly for few days, and then suddenly, at 4.00 am this morning, Martin's pump goes into blaring attention-seeking mode again, indicating that the pump has encountered a blockage. We are shocked out of sleep and into fuddled attempts to determine what has gone wrong and whether it is serious.

A phone call to the Prince Edward doesn't provide any solutions, so Martin is told to turn the pump off and miss his early morning infusion. He is told the nurse will get there first thing in the morning to see what is going on.

We have a somewhat anxious few hours imagining that Martin might have to be readmitted to hospital if the problem is in the PICC line and he has to have another inserted. My personal theory is that the electronics of the pump have been meddled with by the same house gremlins that played with the computer, the mobile phone and the Visa card earlier in the piece. Luckily, however, when the businesslike morning nurse comes to reset the pump's electronics, the gremlins are frightened off and it starts again.

1 September 2009

The magic day is finally here and Martin's IV drip is taken out. No rites to mark the first day of spring could be more joyful. The whole house is lit up with celebratory energy – as if the removal of the drip is the final marker of the passage into health. No more of the medical paraphernalia that singles out the sick person from the well. No more strange beeping at odd times, no more twice-daily visits from the homecare nurse, no more worrying about infected port sites, no more accommodating the inert, extra passenger of the IV container wherever we go. And, most amazingly of all, Martin can now return to dancing.

The last time Martin danced was on the morning of his stroke four months ago. When we venture back onto the dance floor and feel our way back into the steps and sequences, however tentatively, I am near tears – the tears of moved amazement rather than sadness – and I keep seeing, like a split-screen TV, the scenes of Martin paralysed and wordless in June and dancing in September.

The old dances come back easily to him. Many of the newer ones, learned in the months before his stroke, have to be relearned. This would be likely to happen, though, with anyone who has not danced for months. The only thing different that Martin notices is that his timing, which used to be naturally precise, is slightly off. As the weeks go by, however, this normalises, and within months Martin's timing is as effortless as it always was.

Martin has also arranged to start back at his work as a computer analyst. The plan is that he will begin with two days a week and then perhaps move up to three days, which was what he had been doing before the stroke.

He is finding that he can do all the complex, analytical work that he was able to do before the stroke, just not as quickly. Processing takes longer and even simple things like hitting the right keys on the computer slow him down. It is also more tiring – Martin's brain is having to work harder. The things he could do so effortlessly before, he now has to think through and relearn. It takes both time and energy. His keyboard accuracy gets faster with practice, but although he gets back his analytic accuracy, he doesn't get back his previous speed nor the ability to juggle multi-tasking with ease. As Martin worked very speedily pre-stroke, this change of pace, although noticeable to him, probably just places him at around the average speed of performance. And importantly, despite his relative slowing down, he is still able to understand and solve the complex problems that are part of his work.

13 September 2009

Martin is now being monitored as an outpatient by the Prince Edward's Infectious Diseases Unit and the big questions currently on the cards are whether the infection has been killed and what its impact has been on Martin's heart. There is consensus that something is still visible on the various echocardiograms, but opinions, naturally, differ as to what it is. Infectious Diseases is surprised to see anything. Cardiology is surprised that Infectious Diseases is surprised.

Infectious Diseases is investigating the possibility of other disease processes such as lupus and every other illness it can think of as an explanation for the 'something' visible on Martin's mitral valve. Cardiology is sure it is vegetation. And not the chomping kind that cows prefer. Vegetation is the rather charming name for a distinctly uncharming cluster of bacteria.

The big question, if Cardiology is right, is what state is the vegetation in? There are three tickable boxes for this: a) sterile, as in dead and harmless; b) dormant, as in not doing anything right now but might yawn and wake up any moment; and c) alive, as in up and deadly. Which is the correct answer? Roll the dice.

But for the first time in months, Martin's body is his own. He is returning as an outpatient to South-Central Rehab to continue the speech and physio sessions that were abruptly halted with his ambulance ride to the Prince Edward Infectious Diseases Ward. He is back doing his computer work. He can speak, albeit more slowly and with a different accent. And with his return to dancing, he is picking up the piece that was dropped, seemingly shattered, on the dance floor that icy June morning so many centuries ago.

Meanwhile, the multiple tests and investigations are continuing. Each of the various medical departments that claims Martin as its own is proceeding apace with scans and MRIs of various parts of his anatomy.

A couple of weeks ago, it was the turn of the Neurosurgery Department. We sat in the huge, crowded waiting room and waited. For two hours. Each enquiry about when we might be seen was met with a shrug of the shoulders. Despite the fact that Martin's appointment card stated a specific time, it appears this was there only as a sop to the gullible. In fact there is no such thing as a specific time in the timetabling of appointments at the Neurosurgery Clinic. The neurosurgeons and registrars staffing this clinic have clearly achieved the transcendence of the truly evolved spirit – for them time has no existence.

For the less elevated who populate the waiting room, time is very clearly present, and backaches, stress and fatigue increase in exponential relationship to its passage. Although Martin and I can claim all three of the former, as I look around I see people who are far more ill and in more distressing circumstances – they are shockingly frail and in severe pain. And still they have to wait through a whole endless morning.

It has been said that all junior doctors should experience a spell in hospital as a patient before graduating. I would add to that a spell of waiting for hours in hospital waiting rooms, having previously ingested a potion that confers temporary illness and pain and knowing that at the end of this ordeal will come the decision about whether or not they can proceed with their lives.

We are so enveloped in this Kafkaesque limbo that when Martin's name is called at last, we jump in shock. The neurosurgical registrar is a pleasant young man, but the efficiency of interdepartmental communications is living up to familiar standards and the registrar has no idea that Martin has been diagnosed with endocarditis nor that this holds the explanation of what caused his stroke.

'I must write that down', he says, when I inform him.

He schedules another MRI for October to look for any changes to Martin's brain. The swelling will have gone down by then and he wants to see if any abnormalities are revealed.

14 September 2009

In a week, Martin is meeting an OT for his driving assessment – something that is necessary for him to formally reclaim his driver's licence, suspended in the wake of his stroke. Martin is functioning so well that he will cruise through the test and, needless to say, is unbelievably excited about getting back his wheels.

His twice-weekly speech therapy sessions are continuing at South-Central, and at home we are playing as many word games as we can dig up. On walks, we play that old children's stalwart 'I Spy', as well as a variety of 'name the country/person/object starting with a particular letter of the alphabet' games. We have given up on reading the Morecambe and Wise scripts. I never in fact got to find out whether reading humorous scripts out loud was a good way of exercising Martin's speech as we didn't find the *Morecambe and Wise* scripts funny. I turned instead to some John Clarke scripts. They unfortunately proved too funny – we kept cracking up. I am ordering some *Seinfeld* in the hope that they will prove to be the middle-bear of comedy.

1 October 2009

The results from Martin's latest echocardiogram have just come in. The radiologists are still seeing a little 'something' on the mitral valve. Infectious Diseases are still perturbed by this – they don't know whether it is infection or part of the healing process. They are concerned enough to schedule a further echocardiogram in two weeks to see if there are any changes. No one can explain to me why they feel there might be changes in two weeks. Presumably there are only three possibilities: a) it will be smaller or not there (breathe sigh of relief), b) it will be the same (concerned but at least it is not getting worse), or c) it is growing (just panic).

We are left to ruminate on the possibilities and what they might mean until mid-October.

14 October 2009

Martin is about to set out for his repeat echocardiogram. The time, if not the location, was kept top secret. I found out about it only by accident yesterday afternoon when I decided to ring and enquire whether we had been allocated a time slot yet. My phone call was met with puzzlement.

'But you already have one'.

'No one's notified us. Are you sure we have one?'

'I think so. No, wait, let me check some more'.

A dozen back-and-forth phone calls later terminate with the secretary of the Heart Imaging Unit saying to me, 'We'll have to stop meeting this way', and finally confirming that yes we do have an appointment and that no, no one had told us.

I have to hurriedly cancel this morning's patients so that I can be there with Martin. They are obviously worried about the 'something'. During our back-and-forth phone calls, the secretary has informed me that the echo referral is labelled urgent, leaving me in a state of shoved-down panic. If the bug is what they are seeing in Martin's mitral valve and it is alive, Martin is in danger both from the bug damaging his heart and from the possibility of it breaking off again and causing another stroke.

Needless to say, post-scan, the radiologist will not tell us a thing about what she saw – her only comment is that she has to compare this week's image with the previous image and then report to Kathy, the IDU registrar. We are told to ring Kathy on Monday. That is four days of waiting, a time period that in patient life, in a process akin to the calculation of dog years, consists of four months.

It is in fact Tuesday by the time Kathy gets back to us. The echocardiogram was the same as the last one – there is still something there but she still doesn't know what. She doesn't think it is infection, good news, but thinks it might be a clot, bad news. There is also some 'regurgitation'. And no, Martin's heart has not suddenly developed an eating disorder – the term refers to the amount of backwash in the cardiac chambers. Ideally, as the heart pumps blood through its chambers, all of the blood is pushed through in one direction by the heart's valves. When the valves are faulty, not all the blood is pushed on forwards – this is the backwash or regurgitation. When regurgitation is severe, not enough blood is being circulated through the heart and it has to work harder. Eventually its muscles weaken to life-threatening levels and surgery is necessary to save the heart from failing.

Kathy says the regurgitation will have to be monitored and may at some point in the future need surgery to correct it but at the moment is not a problem. However, she adds, the cardiologist will be the expert on this.

Meanwhile, the consultant cardiologist talked to the IDU consultant and decided to do a TOE, the specialised echocardiogram, instead of an ordinary echo. Martin has been saying plaintively to Kathy for a couple of weeks now, 'Why aren't you scheduling a TOE instead of an ordinary echo?'

And, in a surprise move, the Cardiology Clinic rings with an appointment for an actual consultant (so far we have only seen registrars, so we are moving up the hospital phylogenetic scale). Of course, before the consultant cardiologist sees Martin he wants, yes of course, another echocardiogram.

So next week, Martin has another echocardiogram on Tuesday, another MRI on Thursday and, shortly after that, a week where we have a schedule of separate appointments with Cardiology, Neurosurgery and Infectious Diseases. But at least it looks as if by the end of the month we will have some answers.

Update, 22 October 2009

We arrived at today's Infectious Diseases appointment hoping for enlightenment in the wake of Martin's various scans. Alas, answers are apparently not in season. Kathy told us the IDU team's consensus was that the echocardiograms are showing a swinging tag of 'something' on Martin's mitral valve. No one knows what it is and what is causing it. At this point all we, and the doctors, know is that it may or may not be capable of breaking off and causing another stroke, it may or may not be dangerous and, finally, it may or may not be the symptom of yet another disease process. Clearly not the kind of news conducive to calm, untroubled sleep. Martin had seven vials of blood taken and is being tested for everything under the sun. We see the cardiologist in a few days – he is now The Man, as this next round of the game is definitely in Cardiology's court.

A few days before, we had arrived at the Prince Edward for the neurosurgeon's appointment. I had prepared for the usual two-hour wait by packing two novels, a cushion, water, bananas and other assorted picnic paraphernalia. When we checked in at the desk on arrival, the clerk replied tonelessly, 'Two hours', in answer to my wistful query of how long before we would be seen. Fortified by the knowledge that I had two novels with me in case one ran out, I settled down, took out the book and was just about to open it when a doctor popped out of a doorway and called out Martin's name. We had hit the jackpot – a ten-minute wait.

The new MRI looked very different from the old MRI of July. You could see the healing in a very impressive way. In July, Martin's brain was so swollen that the convoluted folds on the outside were almost smooth. Now the wrinkles are back and we can delight in them. Cosmetic ads for the brain would be a startling contrast to their current incarnations for the face. Brain ads would be urging consumers to add more wrinkles. In the brain, wrinkles are good. And more wrinkles are better. The three by three by three-centimetre inkblot covering Martin's expressive speech area where the neurons have died is still there, unchanged. It is astonishing to view it with the knowledge that Martin can now speak and write clearly and well. The extent to which his brain has redesigned itself to accomplish this is both moving and remarkable.

The neurosurgical registrar pronounced herself very pleased with Martin and discharged us from the Neurosurgery Clinic with honours.

Update 21st November 2009

Martin had his TOE on Thursday. The TOE procedure itself seemed only to take about half an hour or so but there was a long wait beforehand and then a two-hour wait afterwards while Martin was monitored to make sure he recovered from the anaesthetic. It is amazing how tiring sitting for six hours in a hospital waiting room can be. Two of the hospital waiting hours *were spent in the company of the blaring daytime-TV talk shows, which I think counts as official torture.*

Martin's TOE turned out to show pretty much what they had expected. The radiologist continued the quirky habit of communicating the technical details of what she saw to a groggy Martin and not communicating them to a not-groggy spouse sitting in the room next door. She instructed Martin to repeat everything to the next person he saw immediately as he would otherwise forget it. Poor Martin started gabbling at a rate of knots the instant he saw me. Upshot is that the radiologist saw exactly the same vegetation as in the ordinary echo – she referred to it as 'dormant' vegetation. I would have preferred to have heard 'dead' vegetation, but time and going off the antibiotics will tell.

Next week we see Kathy in Infectious Diseases and then a couple of weeks after that we see Cardiology again. And this time we are hopeful the planets may have aligned and the two departments might even tell us the same things.

22 November 2009

It is now almost three months since Martin's drip was removed. Investigations aside, he has been feeling well, he is driving, he is back at his computer and he is dancing. We are quietly optimistic. We have passed through the storm. We can take a few breaths.

And that is exactly what we are doing at 10.00 pm on a Sunday evening in late November. We have just returned from a dance class and are happily tired. Martin has sat down to relax for a bit in front of the TV. I have been hanging up my parka in the other room. I come back into the living room to notice Martin seemingly trying to stretch his neck, in the way one does with a mild muscle ache.

'Are you okay?' I ask.

It takes a few seconds for Martin to reply. The movement of his head continues.

'Do you have an ache or an itch?' It still has not dawned on me that this movement is anything out of the ordinary.

Finally Martin speaks. 'I can't stop doing this', he says puzzled.

And my heart drops away. This small repetitive movement is not a scratch or a stretch or an itch or any of the everyday things I want it to be. This is an epileptic seizure.

I have never seen an epileptic fit before but I know enough about them to recognise what is happening. It is not a major one but I am sure this strange, uncontrollable, tic-like motion is a seizure.

'We should get you to the Prince Edward so they can have a look at it', I say, trying to sound calm. My mind is racing around the question of what is causing this – scar tissue from the stroke-injured site or something ominously new stirring into action.

The movement stops after only a minute or so and Martin is conscious, aware and, to all intents and purposes apart from the twitch, his usual self.

'We'll go to the Emergency Department', I say. 'Take a book in case we have to wait a while'. I grab a blanket in the event Martin is left on a stretcher in the sometimes-chilly hospital and we bundle out into the night.

Luckily, traffic is sparse and I drive, alternating concentration on the road with quick sideward glances to check that Martin is still looking normal.

It is ridiculously easy to park outside the Prince Edward, the one advantage of a near-midnight crisis, and we walk through the dark into the bright light of the Emergency Department. It is orderly, organised and remarkably normal-looking. From the odd article I had read about Emergency Department life, I had expected alcohol, blood and aggression, but this Sunday night is demure in its calmness. Sunday night, it seems, is much better timing for medical mishaps than its raucous Saturday sibling.

The triage intake nurse gets to us fairly quickly, and I relate the history of Martin's stroke. One of the registrars will be with us soon, she says, and a CT scan will be organised.

A CT scan, I think to myself, why would they need one of those for a mild epileptic seizure? And then of course I remember what the other possible cause for Martin's symptoms could be – another stroke. That is why they want the CT scan. I say nothing of this to Martin. He seems quite recovered at this stage, his normal self, just puzzled and bemused by his odd, brief experience.

We barely have time to get settled into the waiting room when a registrar ushers us into a cubicle in another section of the unit. There is a gurney there for Martin and he lies down on it, grateful for the woollen rug from home to ward off the chill, against which the thin hospital blankets are helpless. The registrar checks Martin's vital signs, indicates they look okay and says someone will be along soon to take him for his scan. She leaves and I am impressed by the clockwork efficiency.

We settle down expectantly. And then the clockwork runs down. There is activity all around us but none headed in our direction. Martin is yawning and sleepy. We have been closeted in the cubicle for an hour and a half and it is close to midnight. I make attempts to catch the attention of the occasional passing figure but registrars have taken on the elusiveness of taxis on a rain-swept night. Finally, a nurse appears to tell us that a CT scan has been ordered. She tells us this with a 'breaking news' expression that belies the fact another nurse told us this an hour and a half ago. 'When will Martin be having it?' I ask, hoping the breaking news is that it is actually about to happen. She shrugs. 'When they're ready'.

Martin drifts off to sleep. I have done the Boy Scout 'be prepared' thing and brought a book with me. What I have not anticipated is that there will be no light to read by. I have only my chair and myself and a slowed-down sense of time in a setting where time is slowed down already. It is past midnight now, so there is not even the possibility of ringing a friend. Everyone I know will already be asleep. Amantha has a workshop she has to run tomorrow and I have not told her we are at the Prince Edward. There is nothing she can do and she would simply be needlessly stressed. Although I am surrounded by a whole building full of people, I am struck by the feeling of isolation – the imprisoning effect of the midnight hours where all contact with friends is cut off, even through texts or emails.

Another hour crawls by. To the right of us, coming from another cubicle a few metres away a sound has crescendoed above the normal working sounds of the Emergency Department. I have been trying to tell myself it is the sound of machinery. It has the harsh, screechy quality of unceasing grating metal but I am finally forced to admit that it is the sound of human screaming. Unlike most screams, which fluctuate in volume and frequency, this scream has no pauses and no shifts except for the occasional intake of breath. There are no words distinguishable within it, it is just pure…what? Rage? Pain? Fear? Everything primal that terrifies us in the night. The aural transmutation of Munch's art. I keep waiting for someone to attend to the screamer. I peek out of our cubicle but the scream is coming from a curtained area further off. A nurse walks past it without blinking. Is someone looking after the screamer? Has he or she been seen? It is impossible to know. The scream continues unabated throughout the rest of the night.

After another couple of stretched-out hours, the trolley arrives to transport Martin to his CT scan. 'Will it be long before we get the results?' I ask the nurse. I have been hoping to be able to take Martin home to his own bed before the night is over.

'Shouldn't be long', the nurse replies. I fail to notice the 'famous last words' bubble floating above her head.

More time drags by. Martin reappeared from his CT adventure some time ago and is asleep again on his trolley bed. The cubicle is only big enough to accommodate his trolley and the hard plastic chair I am seated on. Martin and I are both early risers – 6.00 am is our normal waking time and by 10.30 pm we are yawning and getting ready for bed. Here, at 3.00 am, my body just wants to cut out, but the chair barely offers basic seating comfort, let alone the ability to stretch out, lean back or curl up. I am astonished by the physical toll that staying awake takes. How many times have I read or heard of people staying awake all night with a relative in hospital and somehow equated it, through the arithmetic of hours, to staying up all day? Night is totally different – your body is desperate to shut itself down, its internal chemistry denying you energy, focus, all the qualities that make up the normal you as you fight to keep awake, make decisions, make assessments, make time pass while the hours stretch like damned versions of Dali's clocks.

The CT results are supposed to have arrived half an hour ago for the last three hours. Each time I enquire I can lip-sync the nurse as she replies, 'They should have been here half an hour ago'. I am therefore startled when on the fourth hourly enquiry the nurse starts with 'They should have' and then abruptly switches to, 'I'll go and check'.

And amazingly she returns. 'There's no radiologist on duty', she announces, 'so no one can read the scans till morning'.

I blink. 'I thought they were supposed to be read hours ago'.

'No'. She shrugs. 'No point in you staying. Your husband's comfortable. Nothing's going to happen till the radiologist gets here at 8.00. You may as well go home and catch some sleep'.

I kiss Martin goodbye and wander in circles for some time before accidentally finding the exit. As I re-enter the house it is close to 4.30 am. Just before I roll onto the bed, still fully clothed, to catch a couple of hours of sleep, I decide to ring the hospital to check that Martin is okay. The nurse in Emergency says 'Ah, yes, Mr Imber. They've just read his scans and they're okay. You can come and pick him up now'.

I drive back in, a little light-headed with the mixture of relief and lack of sleep. Luckily, the traffic is equally light and in fact the most dangerous fellow traveller is a bird, obviously not of the early persuasion, that swoops blearily at the windscreen and swerves off at the last second with a mere centimetre miss.

The word at the Prince Edward is that at this stage they are assuming it is a seizure but they don't know what caused it. They will be making a follow-up appointment with the neurologists and also scheduling an EEG to check on any aberrant electrical behaviour in Martin's brain. And that is it. We are on our way home.

1 December 2009

Our Neurology appointment has been arranged for little more than a week after Martin's seizure – something I fail to recognise at the time as a 'blue moon' phenomenon of speedy scheduling. As usual, I have come prepared with everything we might need to while the afternoon away in the waiting room but, incredibly, we are called in immediately.

The Neurology registrar is very pleasant as he speed-reads through Martin's history. But he is clearly not going to be a fount of wisdom: 'Why didn't they send you to the Stroke Clinic?' he asks, once we have furnished him with the nutshell version of Martin's history since Frankston. Why indeed?

And then, 'Why didn't they get the Neurology registrar on call to see you in the Emergency Department that Sunday night?'

And when I ask him what the frequency of seizures is in the months post-stroke, he rubs his chin and says with musing and disarming candour, 'I must ask my colleagues in the Stroke Department about that'.

In between the shrugging, he organises an EEG for a week's time, which he expects to be normal, and a return appointment in a month. The impression we get is that it is not a big deal. It is not a stroke, there is no further damage to Martin's brain, it was just a blip – a buzz of errant electricity zipping through Martin's brain. Just a hiccup.

His cheerful parting words are, 'You really should have been sent to the Stroke Unit, but we'll have to do instead'.

10 December 2009

Today we have Cardiology on our minds. Although there have been a series of echocardiograms since Martin's stroke, the reports from each have been reassuring. Despite the fact that 'something' is visible on the mitral valve of the heart, Martin's heart function looks reasonable – the endocarditis has managed not to wreak any major damage. There is some regurgitation, but it is mild and manageable and will not require any intervention.

The multiple investigations launched by Infectious Diseases to discover the nature of the 'something' on Martin's mitral valve have come back negative. A lot of very nasty diseases have been ruled out. And we have been told several times that Martin's heart is working well enough to mean surgery will not be required.

We are so complacent about this in fact that we are relaxed and smiling in the cardiologist's waiting room, joking to each other that we are actually getting to see a Prince Edward consultant this morning instead of the usual registrar – a move akin to scoring first-class seats on the plane instead of sardine class. We are being upgraded.

The consultant, Dr D., greets us cordially. His first question is 'Who ordered all these repeat echocardiograms?' As we have been told that it was Dr D. who had ordered all these repeat echocardiograms, we look slightly mystified.

He digs the echo out of a pile of paper on his desk, eyeballs it and pronounces confidently that there are two patches on the mitral valve (the 'swinging tag' Kathy has been seeing has suddenly become two patches when viewed with Dr D. vision) and that it was clearly vegetation. He then launches straight into his opinions on Infectious Diseases' various investigations: 'The echo shows some vegetation on your mitral valve and it's clear that's what it is. If it barks like a dog and looks like a dog, it is a dog. No idea why Infectious Diseases is investigating all these other things'.

'Is it possible the vegetation is from an infection that's still active?' I ask.

'Might be', he says nonchalantly. 'Only real way to tell is if it flares up again'. He pauses and then adds with equal nonchalance, 'And of course, there's a very high chance of that happening'.

And just as we are digesting that statement, he launches into the real bombshell – the damage to Martin's mitral valve is not minor. It has grown up, got its driver's licence and voting rights, and has qualified as a definite major. The kind of major that will require surgery. Delicate, complex open-heart surgery.

With our jaws still metaphorically touching the floor, Dr D. continues apace. He is sure, he says, that Martin will not be a candidate for a mitral valve repair. Instead, he will have to have a mitral valve replacement and, with mitral valves, replacements have to be metal. For Martin, this is especially problematic, as bugs prefer to nest on metal rather than tissue. Because Martin's heart has already been bug-infested, he is at an especially high risk of further infection with a metal valve replacement. And, Dr D. re-emphasises cheerily, Martin is at high risk anyway, even without the metal valve, for recurrences of heart infection. In fact, Dr D. gathers even more enthusiasm here, Martin is bound to have another heart infection. Then, as the cherry on the cake, he chattily confides to us that very few surgeons do mitral valve operations and that they are particularly difficult surgeries to perform.

He tells us he will order another monitoring echocardiogram in three months and that we shouldn't delay too long in having the surgery. He then stares at us wordlessly in the sympathetic manner of a practised undertaker.

We recover ourselves for the usual polite automatic thankyous one gives on these occasions. Dr Doom, as I am starting to think of him, has been so full of 'absolutes' and 'definites' there is no room for questions. We make the pre-getting-up shuffling motions of reaching for bags and coats.

At this point he is supposed to play his part in the leaving ritual and stand to usher us out. Instead, he remains seated, staring at us fixedly and mournfully as if in the presence of great tragedy.

Politely, we remain seated. 'Thank you', we say again, 'you've explained everything'.

More minutes go by. Not the politely waiting minutes of 'any questions?' but the awkward silence of someone faced with the bereaved and not knowing how to end the contact. It is intensely creepy.

Finally, he rouses himself, stands and ushers us out.

Martin and I walk down the corridor dulled with shock. Each time we think we are heading out of the woods, the giant hand from comic books and advertising campaigns has picked us up and dumped us back in.

Dr Doom's words have taken up residence in my brain with a density approaching that of matter in black holes. Their weight feels as if it is compressing my body by actual inches, slowing down my physical self as well as my thinking.

There is a disease known to affect snakes in captivity. The media calls it mad-snake disease but its technical name is 'inclusion body disease'. It strikes pythons and boa constrictors. Affected snakes display strange behaviours, such as 'stargazing' – staring endlessly, aimlessly upwards, with a drunken-seeming inability to coordinate themselves. In their confused writhing, they eventually tie themselves into knots from which they cannot untangle themselves, their movements devolving slowly into a final knotted stasis. I am reminded of this now as we move, seemingly in slow motion and near wordlessly, down the corridor, our brains in the 'stalled' mode, trying to reposition reality.

By the time we get to the car, my brain starts functioning again. Dr Doom said that surgeons who perform mitral valve surgeries are rare. I am not a cardiologist but that makes no sense to me. Valve replacements and repairs have to be common surgical needs among cardiac patients. Why would mitral valve repairs be any less frequent than aortic valve repairs? Along with coronary artery bypass surgery, they must be one of the most requested and necessary procedures. It has to be something a lot of cardiac surgeons are expert in. I am sure of this. It must be nonsense to say that few cardiac surgeons have the expertise to operate on the mitral valve. What other 'facts' with which Dr Doom has presented us are also false?

I get home and start contacting friends to get the name of a good cardiologist. We need an opinion other than Dr Doom's. Unfortunately, it is nearing Christmas, so getting a cardiologist appointment is like getting special entree an hour ahead of the crowds for the post-Christmas sales. Finally, after hours of phone calls, I strike it lucky – a cancellation has just freed up a space in the office of one of the recommended cardiologists.

We are as excited as if we have won the lottery. We need this new specialist. We need someone to do the American Indian smoke cleansing thing, speak the magic syllables, mix up the voodoo potions that will rid us of the lingering weight of Dr Doom's predictions.

15 December 2009

We are back at the Prince Edward today for Martin's EEG, organised as a result of his mini-seizure. We walk past the familiar terrain of his old alma mater, 5 West , the Neurology Ward – distinguishable as usual not only by the signs, but by the anguished, continual screams coming from one of the beds.

While Martin is occupied with the EEG, I race around the Prince Edward – upstairs and downstairs and everywhere but my lady's chamber, in an effort to get Martin's medical records. Our appointment with the private cardiologist tomorrow becomes meaningless without Martin's accompanying health records.

I pant my way around the hospital, attempting to locate the records – the fourth floor, the second floor, the first floor, the third floor and back to the second floor. Having finally located them, the next labour is to wrest them from the safekeeping of the Cardiology Department's dragons. I brandish my letter of permission from Martin, explaining that I had talked to the freedom of information people yesterday and they had assured me that all I had to do was come in and pick them up. No dice. The supervisor regards me as if I were a criminal mastermind attempting to snatch the Hope diamond. Finally, after much negotiation, she allows me to take a sealed envelope with the written reports, reiterating that on *no account* am I allowed to open it. She refuses point-blank, however, to give me a copy of the CT films.

I go back to the EEG unit, ring the freedom of information people and have a lengthy discussion with them on the meaning of the Freedom of Information Act. It seems the main purpose of the Freedom of Information Act is to make it as difficult as possible for patients to access their own records.

Martin emerges, having just finished the EEG proceedings, as I get off the phone.

'Any hints about what they saw?' I ask. But of course there are none – we will have to wait until our appointment with the Neurology Department next week to get the results.

17 December 2009

Today we have our appointment with Dr R., the new private cardiologist. He is calm and competent, examines Martin thoroughly and dispels Dr Doom's pronouncements on the rarity of mitral valve operations. As I had surmised, valve replacements and repairs are part of the bread and butter of cardiac surgeons, and mitral valve surgeries are as common as those involving the aortic valves.

Dr R. orders another echo in early January and will get the rest of Martin's records from the Prince Edward, see us in a couple of weeks and tell us what he thinks, although he is fairly sure that cardiac surgery is in Martin's future. He does say, though, that he would be very wary of recommending surgery while there was any chance the endocarditis was dormant rather than dead. This we will not know until Martin goes off the antibiotics and is closely monitored for any signs of returning infection.

21 December 2009

It is back to Infectious Diseases. Last time we saw Kathy, the IDU registrar, she said this appointment would mark the time for Martin to go off his antibiotics and see what happens. Not surprisingly, this is what we are expecting to hear when the appointment comes up.

Big mistake. As we are rapidly finding out, going into an appointment with any expectation is simply the equivalent of sending out a gilt-edged invitation signed by Mr and Mrs Hubris and addressed to Fate.

And sure enough, when we turn up to this session, the new consensus decision is in fact to keep Martin on the antibiotics. This bug is known to be a recidivist – it has a tendency to come back and Infectious Diseases are worried that if Martin comes off treatment now, it may do just that.

I mention that Dr R., the cardiologist, has said he wouldn't recommend surgery until Martin has been off the antibiotics and follow-up has shown no sign of the bug resurfacing, Kathy looks a little puzzled. 'You'd have to go on the antibiotics pre-surgery anyway', she says, 'so why go off them?' We shrug. In some perfect universe, consultants from the different specialties actually talk to each other.

22 December 2009

It is time to get the results of Martin's EEG. We are anxious, but not overly so, as we enter one of the Neurology consulting rooms. After all, the Neurology registrar expected the EEG results to be normal. The epileptic fit was so mild and localised it could barely count as a fit. Surely?

It is a pleasant surprise to see a professor sitting behind the desk instead of the usual registrar. Our upgrading at the Prince Edward is on a steep curve. From a registrar to a consultant to a professor.

The professor is a man I have heard of, with a reputation for decency as well as great expertise. He is calm, warm and respectful but his news is not what we want to hear. Abnormalities have indeed shown up in Martin's EEG. The problem is the wrong mix of Greek letters. Too many delta waves where there should have been betas and alphas.

The wave patterns showing up are indicating an area of damage that has been caused by scar tissue from the stroke. And seizures starting a few months after a stroke, as opposed to those start-ing immediately after, are highly likely to continue. There is a small chance, he says that this might be an isolated one, but it is highly unlikely.

Given that there is a small chance, however, we can have a choice – start on anti-epileptic medication immediately or take the chance that it will not happen again and delay starting on medication. But whichever choice we make, Martin will not be allowed to drive for at least six months. Martin's face falls at this news. Although the Emergency Department registrar had not forbidden driving, we had talked with Martin's new GP and he had suggested not driving for three months. Martin had been counting off the weeks. To have his sentence doubled is a blow for him – his driving is his independence and it has been a joy for him in recent weeks to have been allowed back behind the wheel.

Just before we leave, the professor adds that the seizure Martin experienced was a very mild one, classified as a partial, simple seizure. If he does go on to have further seizures, it is likely they will be more major ones. This is a sobering thought, but we go for optimism and decide we will forgo medication for the moment in the hope this episode will prove an isolated incident.

As the door of the professor's office closes behind us, we progress down the hospital corridors in the usual stunned post-consultative state.

4 January 2010

Martin's umpteenth echocardiogram finally comes through and we have our second appointment with our new cardiologist, Dr R., to get the results. Basically January's results are the same as December's – that is, moderate to severe regurgitation in the mitral valve. The even earlier July report had noted only mild regurgitation, so there has been a deterioration between July and December. Dr R. is still saying that a 'watch and wait' approach would be best, however. He says that as long as there is no further deterioration, there is no pressing need for surgery, and as the surgery is a major assault on the body, there is no need to rush to it unless absolutely necessary. He tells us to watch out for any signs of deterioration.

'Does deterioration happen gradually?' I ask.

'Yes', he answers. 'Unless it happens suddenly'.

'Do you have an estimate of a time line?' I ask.

He makes the universal 'anyone's guess' gesture – it could happen tomorrow or it could happen years from now.

I then ask about the risks of waiting. He replies but somehow doesn't answer the question. And then the appointment is over. He suggests another echo and review four months from now.

But the timing of the surgery keeps bugging me. In Dr R.'s view, delaying the operation and simply 'watching and waiting', even for years, doesn't risk extra deterioration of the heart muscles. I cannot make sense of this. We know a chorda has ruptured in Martin's mitral valve, so mechanical stress is being placed on the heart – and anything mechanical, out of balance and in constant motion must be highly likely to worsen over time, as different parts take on strains and stresses they are not designed for. The more deterioration in the valve the less chance Martin has of getting the needed repair instead of the more problematic replacement valve. Surely, then, operating later rather than earlier has to have some risks attached to it.

Back home, I summon Dr Google and dig out a couple of meta-studies comparing the outcomes of early surgery with 'watch and wait' on asymptomatic severe mitral valve regurgitation, and they show that early surgery has a better outcome than watching and waiting. I don't know it yet, but in three years' time a definitive study on this question will be released. A study led by the Mayo Clinic will challenge the long-held belief that it is safer to watch and wait until the patient has symptoms. The results of the study show that early surgery for severe mitral valve regurgitation gives significantly better results than watching and waiting. The sooner the surgeon can plug up the leak, ideally with a mitral valve repair, the better for the patient's long-term health. Patients who had surgery within three months of diagnosis did better than those who delayed surgery for more than three months following diagnosis.

But I don't know this yet. All I have at the moment is my own unease and the handful of smaller studies I have been able to find. Matched against the expert judgement of two consultant cardiologists, who have been unable to explain to me why they are choosing the watch-and-wait path they are suggesting.

It is becoming clear that we are between a rock and a hard place – Scylla and Charybdis and all those other competing, deadly and well-matched sets of options. No one is going to give us the definitive 'This is what you must do' instruction, but at least now I know the right questions to ask. And I want to understand the answers. Time to find a third cardiologist.

9 January 2010
Multiple enquiries eventually throw up the name of a cardiologist recommended by three people I trust. And, miracle of miracles, we have actually scored an appointment. It is tomorrow and I have meticulously prepared my list of questions, got everything organised for the morning and have just gone into the bedroom to get my shoes for our evening of dancing. I return to the living room after an absence of a moment and Martin is sitting on the couch and his head is convulsively twitching.

I run over and hold him. 'Are you okay?' I say, in that utterly useless phrase we all use when everything is clearly not okay.

But this time Martin cannot answer. His eyes are open, but he is not there. The twitch has turned into spasms and galloped from just his neck to his whole body. He is making terrible inhuman sounds. He is having a full-blown epileptic fit.

In the future, whenever I talk to people about epilepsy, the first thing I will ask is 'Have you ever seen someone have an epileptic fit?' And if they say no, I know they can never understand.

I of course think I have seen epileptic fits before – on TV shows, where the disease-to-be-detected sometimes involves an actor having a fit. I have read descriptions of epileptic fits. I thought I knew what an epileptic fit was. But I have had no idea.

Watching someone you love, or know, have an epileptic fit in front of you is a world away from watching one on TV, reading about it or hearing about it. Just as we find it hard to imagine our own death, it is equally hard to imagine the mini-death, even if we know it is temporary, of the self while the body is still violently active and clearly not asleep. It is horrifying to witness. The body is wickedly animated and alive, but where is the person?

The ancients, of course, had their own answer. The self has been driven out by demons. And as I try to steady Martin's flailing limbs and reassure him, even though he cannot hear me, and helplessly fail to stop him from falling to the floor, where, he bucks and jerks like a mad, animated scarecrow, I can understand, I can totally understand, why the ancients were so terrified.

It seems like an hour but it is only a handful of minutes before the jerks start to diminish and then finally cease. Martin mutters something incoherent and attempts to rise, even though he cannot.

'Wait', I say. 'Just rest for a few minutes'.

But he cannot understand and tries to push me out of the way. He is panting like a marathon runner, sweat pouring down his face. With the uncoordinated movements of a toddler and a lot more strength, he pushes himself upwards, determined to rise and get somewhere. He half gets there and I manage to catch him before he falls again. He is frantic to get to his feet, fighting me off with inarticulate grunts.

Finally, I persuade him to lie down on the carpet, with a cushion for his head and slowly, very slowly, he starts to get some words and orientation back. He has no memory of what has happened. His last memory was his neck starting to twitch and then nothing. I explain to him what has happened. He takes it in.

'How are you feeling?' I ask.

He is still finding it hard to form words. 'Exhausted', he manages.

And I have to decide what to do. If I take him into the Prince Edward, I know we will end up missing tomorrow's precious appointment with our new, new cardiologist. Another one will take months to come along. The Prince Edward had said, in response to my query last time, that it is usually not necessary to take someone into hospital after an epileptic fit. 'Usually', that wonderfully indeterminate word. And no one mentioned that an epileptic fit would leave Martin lost for language again. Could it mean that there is more damage to his brain? Might it be necessary after all to take him to the Prince Edward?

I have no idea. But I have to decide. Martin is pale, spent, but back to consciousness. His body is responding normally again even though he is still fumbling for words. I reason to myself that an electrical storm in the area damaged by the stroke would be likely to disrupt his verbal functioning. And if it is a temporary effect of the epileptic fit, there is no point in hospitalisation, scans and so on. And we have to keep tomorrow's cardiology appointment. And so I put Martin to bed and spend a good deal of the rest of the night shivering with shock and all of it on hyper-alert for every smallest movement or sound.

30 January 2010

This morning, I discover that all of my leg and thigh muscles feel as if I have been running up fifty flights of stairs, a result of all the muscular contractions in last night's violent shivering. I realise I have discovered the next new marketing miracle in lower-body muscle-toning: 'Train in your own bed in your own time. No gym membership required. Just give yourself a hell of a shock beforehand, head off to bed and voilà'. I also discover that each time I walk into the living room I get an involuntary, terrible flashback to Martin's body jerking and convulsing.

Martin has slept through the night and by next morning is feeling tired but back to himself, although he is slower in finding words and finds speaking more difficult than before the fit. It is clear now that he will have to go onto the anti-epileptic medication. With naive optimism, I ring the Prince Edward to make a speedy appointment. The speediest the Prince Edward can manage, it turns out, is a month away. I explain the situation but Neurology is all booked out. Luckily I manage to get an appointment with Martin's GP in the afternoon and, luckier still, I can remember the name of the drug the professor had suggested Martin try first, Tegretol.

In the meantime, there is our much-needed new, new cardiologist's appointment this morning. I have my usual list of questions typed out, along with a précis of Martin's post-stroke medical history and the echo reports. It is like preparing for a business meeting. Peter, the cardiologist, ushers us in warmly and listens to Martin tell his story. As he examines Martin, he asks him what it feels like for him to speak and find words. He is not asking these questions clinically – they are, after all, not symptoms that concern his specialty – he is asking out of a genuine sense of interest. He says to Martin, 'I can see you're a person of real determination who works hard at things'. And I nearly fall out of my chair. He is seeing Martin as a person! Throughout our parade of specialist medicos – some competent, some incompetent, some warm, some cool, no one has stopped to think about Martin as an individual human being or what the interior experience of his illness has been like.

Examination over, Peter concurs that Martin's mitral valve does indeed have significant damage and will require surgery. The surgery doesn't have to happen tomorrow but it will have to happen. I ask my question about the pros and cons of waiting versus jumping in and he answers it clearly and comprehensively. Essentially, he says that waiting a few months longer will mean Martin's brain will have had a year since the stroke to settle down and it will also give the epilepsy a chance to be stabilised – both good things in open-heart surgery, which involves major stresses to the body. He suggests doing a stress echocardiogram (a cardiogram taken after strenuous exercise) as an extra monitoring measure to keep track of how Martin's heart is functioning. Sometimes stress echoes will come up with different numbers to the normal echo. The stress echo results will help us pick the right timing for the surgery and he suggests alternating stress echoes with normal echoes over the next months.

This is a new piece of information – the other two cardiologists have not even mentioned the possibility of stress echoes, but of course it makes sense. The stressed heart and the resting heart may be functioning at different levels. A cardiologist who thinks about stress echocardiograms, explains things, answers questions clearly, and responds to Martin as a person – I am in heaven. We have found our cardiac home.

Peter, of course, doesn't realise this, and when he has concluded, he says mildly, 'Now, you've been to two other senior cardiologists. I know them and I know they would give you the same opinions about this as I have and also the same management program?'

And the question mark on the end of his sentence has its own sentence – it says 'Why three?' the subtext being 'Are you desperate doctor-shoppers who are looking for an impossible response? Are you hypercritical perfectionists for whom nothing is good enough? Are you chasing the fantasy of an ideal doctor who doesn't exist?' He is looking mildly perturbed.

And I rush to reassure him. With all the fervour of Olivia Newton-John singing to John Travolta, I say hurriedly, 'You're the one that we want'.

He raises an eyebrow slightly.

'No one else has suggested a stress echo', I say. 'No one else has answered our questions so clearly, and no one else has explained why they're choosing the management plan they've suggested and what the pros and cons are. That's what we were looking for. We're really happy with this session and we want to stay with you'. And I have to restrain myself from adding 'please'.

Peter nods. 'Okay', he says.

And we are on. We are a therapeutic partnership. And as we go on, he will put John Travolta in the shade – he is definitely the one that we want.

After Peter's session we move on to our afternoon doctor *de jour*, who is also worthy of being sung to. Martin's new GP, Robert, is wonderful – thorough, intelligent, kind and expert. Martin has become his patient only recently. Until then he was without a GP, and throughout the past months of his stroke and endocarditis, I have had to micro-manage everything myself. That has meant, as well as the usual tasks of looking up research and understanding which questions need to be asked, working out which specialist doctors are best and managing the oxymoronic intercommunication between specialists, as well as collating and making sense of their various pronouncements. It is a huge relief to have a GP who can manage the bread and butter of Martin's medical needs and suggest the best referrals instead of the endless 'Do you know a good specialist in [tick the appropriate box]?' phone calls I have had to make to friends.

One of the tick-the-appropriate-box specialists we have decided to find is in neurology and specifically stroke medicine. The name that has risen to the top is that of Elizabeth. Unfortunately, her earliest appointment is a few months away. I have rung that morning to see if there is any way we can get an earlier appointment but all we are offered is an appointment with someone junior in the same practice.

'If we start off with him, can we shift to Elizabeth in March?' I ask. And the answer is no, the practice doesn't work that way. So it is decision time again. Do we go with someone less experienced so that Martin can be seen sooner, or do we wait so that we can get the most senior? I decide we will wait. Martin's new turn with epilepsy is frightening, it needs treating but it is not a medical emergency.

But this afternoon at Martin's appointment, Robert simply picks up the phone and rings Elizabeth to check that she would go with Tegretol too. And I am struck again by the access, and with it power, that doctors have. The knowledge of how medical systems work, the ability to pick up a phone and be responded to, the friends in the right places. The rest of us are immigrants, abruptly and unwillingly deposited in a country with a foreign tongue, unknown customs and a power structure inaccessible, ineluctable and absolute.

And so I go home to consult with 'I talk to everyone' Dr Google. Egalitarian as he is, Dr Google is not comforting. A number of medical sites explain epilepsy, but they are not the ones I am drawn to – I already know the medical information they contain. What I want to know about are the anti-epileptic medications. Do they work and what do they feel like? What are their side effects? I turn to the discussion forums.

Bad idea. Every forum I read is full of people detailing crippling side effects and failing treatments. They fill me with horror. There is a range of medications available for epilepsy – many of them I recognise from their other usage as psychiatric drugs – but for every one that I look up, there is the rather bland official clinical description and, alongside it, the patients' descriptions of unrelieved grogginess, headaches, depression, minimal energy, inability to concentrate and a host of other equally unpleasant side effects.

I am stopped in my tracks. I have always, with a naivety that smacks of denial, thought of medicine as what you take to stop unpleasant symptoms. Somehow, despite the fact that during my ovarian cancer days I have been the recipient of six months of chemotherapy, I have never visualised a future in which the medicine you take for life, as opposed to the mere months of a chemotherapy series, is going to make you feel well and truly sick. And of course there are so many illnesses for which this is true – the cocktail of drugs AIDS patients need to ingest, the immunosuppressors of transplant patients, the ongoing chemo regimes of long-term cancer patients. And now, of course, for the illness that is going to hit close to home – the anti-epileptic medications.

I say nothing of this to Martin. Oddly enough, throughout all of these months, Martin has felt basically well. Apart from the initial grogginess and confusion in the first few days after his stroke, he has had no headaches, pain or nausea. He has been aware of, and terribly frustrated by, his speech problems and the initial paralysis of his arm, but he has been clear-headed and pain-free – an extraordinary blessing.

Like many of us, Martin is not good at being sick – when he gets a cold, he gets a 'man cold'. His usual calm self dissolves into a Mr Hyde-esque double, with all the brooding and irritability that go with it. I cannot imagine what having to tolerate the side effects so vividly described by Dr Google's correspondents would do to him.

But I am about to find out. The Tegretol is an innocuous-looking pill, but its effect on Martin is major. A few hours after taking it, Martin is sitting slumped at the kitchen table, thoroughly and utterly miserable. He is groggy, dizzy and nauseous, says he cannot think straight and that everything feels foggy and leaden. It is an effort to drag him out for a walk in the sunshine.

I remind him that the side effects diminish after a couple of weeks and that within a few days he is likely to be feeling a lot better. He nods weakly. I have to stop myself launching into a buck-up pep talk – the urgency of which is fuelled by the words I have left unspoken 'What if the side effects don't diminish?' I am looking at Martin now, slumped, miserable, down in the deepest of dumps, and I am seeing the future – years and years of this – and I cannot bear it. It seems the cruellest of ironies to have gone through all we have gone through – all the indignities and disabilities against which Martin has so determinedly fought back – to be felled by this.

I swallow all this down and organise Martin on the couch, where he is too lethargic to even watch TV.

'Give it another couple of days', I say and head upstairs like a moth to its fatal flame, in a vain effort to find someone on one of those forums who has not had a ghastly experience with anti-epileptic drugs.

3 February 2010

After three and half days of Tegretol Martin could tolerate no more. He rang his GP who said to wait a day and then start on a new drug, Epilim. At sixteen hours post-Tegretol, Martin is smiling again. It is such a relief to see him back to his normal self.

And then, miracle of miracles, we get a cancellation spot with our hoped-for new neurologist, Elizabeth. She has a terrific reputation and is at the top of her field – it will be wonderful to be in the hands of an expert. And that phrase 'be in the hands of' is so deeply true. What it brings is the experience of being held. Just as for many of us when we first learned to swim, we were held and supported in that strange new element, so too in the frightening, foreign territory of serious illness do we also yearn to be held. To be supported and guided by someone experienced. Someone capable, who knows what to do.

4 February 2010

Elizabeth turns out to be just what we need – pleasant, super-competent and able to answer all our questions. The answers, of course, are not exactly what we want to hear, but they are clear. The fact that Martin's seizure is of late onset post-stroke means he will have to be on anti-epileptic meds for life. Elizabeth is also ordering an MRI on the off-chance that the seizure was a stroke caused by further bits of bug floating loose. Martin is on his second day of Epilim, and although he has been feeling a little bit off in the morning, he is feeling better by the afternoon. I ask Elizabeth what the half-life of Tegretol is and she says it is possible that some of it may still be moving out of his system, explaining his improvement from morning to afternoon.

Then, of course, we are on to the question of when Martin should schedule his heart surgery. I ask Elizabeth her opinion from a neurological standpoint and she says sooner rather than later. The cardiologist prefers later rather than sooner, and in a couple of weeks, when we have an appointment with the Infectious Diseases Unit, we will get a chance to see what they think about the timing – undoubtedly middling as we play Goldilocks and the Three Specialists.

What they are all unanimously saying, though, is that the last thing Martin needs in his system is a replacement heart valve, due to the bug's preference for metal over tissue. As the mitral version comes only in metal, a repair rather than a replacement has become our current desperate wish.

11 February 2010

Faith, the dear friend who was overseas at the time of Martin's stroke, has been back home for a few months now. She arrived back in July, just a few weeks after Martin's stroke. She and I have talked on the phone but I still have not seen her. Faith and the man she fell in love with a few years ago got married last year, and he has decided to move from the United Kingdom, where he has been living and working, to live in Australia with her. I know they have been busy, but when three months tick past and Faith still has not found time for that cup of tea and a hug, I wonder if something is wrong – this is so uncharacteristic of her.

I ring to check that all is well with her. She is flourishing - loving being with her husband and enjoying the full calendar of cultural and social engagements that is standard for her.

'Yes', she says, when I say I would love that cup of tea and catch-up. 'I'll ask Gabe if I can take a couple of hours away from him'.

'You'll ask Gabe?' I say. Faith is a 71-year-old independent, professional woman who has been shaping her own life for decades.

'Yes', she says. 'He's new to the country'.

Faith's response is unusual but she sounds fine and we agree she will get back to me with a time to get together.

And time goes on. We talk on the phone regularly and Faith sounds just the same as her usual self, but nearly half a year has now gone by and we still have not seen each other. Throughout three decades of close and loving friendship, we have been there for each other in whatever circumstances we have encountered. We both lead busy lives but we have always made space for each other. Faith lives only twenty minutes away, and for her to have not once made the time to see a dear friend during a period of such major health crises is unheard of.

I have known Faith when she was single, married, divorced, single and partnered again. I have known her through her busy full-time psychotherapy practice and through her retirement. We have known each other through life-threatening illness, through the death of parents, through experiences of every flavour. For all the time I have known her, she has always been deeply and authentically herself, always totally true to her core values. And those values are embedded in every part of Faith's life – compassion, spirituality, honesty, loyalty and an openness and commitment to discussion and enquiry.

Faith and I met decades back at a week-long residential conference for therapists. Amid the forty odd participants, we stumbled upon each other by accident. We shared a love of poetry, myth and dream; a similarly intuitive approach to working with psychological issues; core values that resonated; and a deep appreciation of each other's hearts and minds. We quickly grew close and have maintained that closeness without exception over the years.

Faith and I have always been open with each other. We have always felt known by the other. For the first time in thirty years of deep and intimate friendship, I am suddenly encountering a Faith who is unfamiliar to me.

I tell her that I am puzzled and a little hurt that we still have not managed to have that cup of tea and hug. Again, Faith says she will ask Gabe when she can take some time.

The weeks pass and then finally, nearly seven months after Martin's stroke, Faith makes a time to meet. And by now I am feeling genuinely concerned. This meeting will be more than our usual cup of tea and hug; I feel as if I need to understand what is happening, who this new Faith is.

On the morning of our meeting, I find an email from Faith in my in-box. She says she has a severe sinus infection, splitting headaches, sore eyes and a mountain of work. It is clear to me that this is not the best time to be having an in-depth conversation.

I email back that it doesn't make sense for her to drive out here when she is feeling so sick, that it would be better for her to rest. We can make another time to see each other.

Faith interprets my suggestion that she rest at home as anger.

I reply that I was motivated not by anger but by sheer practicality, and that I am looking forward to meeting when she is well and has time.

And more weeks go by. Finally, it is eight months since we have seen each other. Faith is included in my daily group-update list and she responds regularly via email. The voice in the emails is the same loving and caring Faith I have known for so long. But in the times we get to speak on the phone, she varies. Sometimes she sounds like the old Faith. Mostly she sounds different in a way that is hard to categorise.

She agrees that we are long overdue for that cup of tea and again says she will ask Gabe about taking a couple of hours out for it. She will contact me with a time to meet and talk.

I am relieved that we are going to meet at last. I have been mystified by this shift in Faith and I want to understand what is happening. I know that what we have to talk through will likely stir up emotions, but we have always been able to talk to each other about anything. We are both psychotherapists – we have never been afraid of complexity or emotion.

I am imagining that when we meet we will either be able to fully reconnect and resume our friendship or that Faith will say that she cannot find the space in her life right now and ask for time out, a sabbatical, before she is free to reconnect. The latter is not my first preference, of course, but it will be manageable. I trust in the strength of our connection to each other. It can withstand time apart, even if it is not the timing I would wish it to be. Our friendship is too precious simply to discard at the first sign of trouble. We care deeply about each other, and it is worth sacrifice and compromise. I am very clear on this and prepared to accept the sabbatical if that is what Faith needs. But I do need this face-to-face meeting – to be able to really communicate, to hug each other and to cross the bridge that has been separating us these last months.

I am expecting to hear from Faith to organise a time to get together and I do hear from her. The message comes in a card delivered via the post. It says quite simply: 'I have been thinking deeply and carefully about our conversations over the past months and come to the painful conclusion that I cannot maintain our friendship'.

I have been fired by post.

The shock is stunning. My first response is disbelief – it is so bizarre that it is not true. I re-read the letter. It is true.

Apart from its impossible-to-take-in content, this dismissal, which comes with such finality, such unilaterality, without the chance to talk, is made even more extraordinary by the fact that

Faith is a psychotherapist who believes in talking things through. Ending a mere acquaintanceship in this way would be atypical for Faith. To end a deep, thirty-year relationship with a beloved friend by this method is unimaginable for the Faith I knew. It is made even more baffling in that we have not had a falling-out, not even an argument.

There are some friendships for which a plunge into life-threatening crisis would have proved fatal in and of itself. Many people who have gone through intense crises have discovered that certain friends simply disappear. I have heard these stories time and time again. I have experienced it in my own life with my two cancer diagnoses. In *Eating the Underworld* I wrote about the shock of finding that two close friends to whom I had given sustained support over the years became furious and raged at me when I was diagnosed with a recurrence and was asking for some support instead of giving it. A third close friend, to whom I had also given a great deal of support, simply disappeared and never reappeared.

Those experiences forced me to look into myself and recognise my own part in those relationships. I have always been someone who takes care of people. In much younger days, it was a part of how I understood my role in the world. I felt qualified to give. I didn't feel entitled to ask – that was the message I unconsciously sent out. My illnesses became a turning point for me in thinking about friendships and taking responsibility for what I needed within them.

I have some wonderful friends, both old and new, and I know that I can turn to all of them for help just as they can turn to me. And Faith and I have always been like that – truly reciprocal in our relationship. Through all manner of lows as well as highs, we have been steadfastly there for each other, cheering each other through our successes and supporting each other through difficult times. Neither of us is a high-maintenance friend – we don't need tiptoeing around or excessive 'feeding'. We have stayed secure in our place in each other's hearts through a variety of conditions. I had imagined that this was how it would always be.

I write back in response to Faith's card, telling her of my shock and sadness on receiving it. I say that I had thought she might want to take time out from our friendship until she had more space for it and that I would have been able to accept that and feel secure in our ability to pick it up again when the time was right.

But she doesn't reply.

And so, in the midst of all the ongoing stress and uncertainty around Martin's health, I find myself on the express train, visa in hand, to the unexpected country of disenfranchised grief.

There are many griefs and losses in our lives that are recognised and stamped by our culture as 'legitimate' – death, divorce, life-threatening illness. We understand that they are 'worthy' griefs – losses that by their weightiness demand an appropriate response, whether we are able to give it or not. They are quite literally card-carrying griefs, as any visit to a greeting-card stand will affirm.

There are just as many griefs that, although similarly painful, are deemed unworthy of this recognition. They are the losses for which there is no condolence card. Losses that are brushed off. Losses deemed too 'minor' to warrant sustained sympathy. Losses that make people uncomfortable. Losses no one wants to talk about, that are kept safely out of sight.

Among the more common of these are losses through miscarriage, abortion, the loss of a family home, the loss of a job, the death of a pet, the break-up of a secret relationship, the child lost to a drug habit, the losses of botched cosmetic surgery, the estrangement of family members, the pain of the mother who gives her child up for adoption, the distress that an ex-spouse's remarriage can bring, the heartache of the infertile couple who long for children. The list goes on.

And taking its place among these disenfranchised griefs is the loss of a best friend. This particular loss comes with its own ten extra steak knives. The person to whom you would naturally turn for support at a time of loss, your best friend, is in fact the person you have lost.

Friendships come and go throughout our lives, of course. Often they die in a drifting-apart manner due to factors such as geographic separation, the development of different interests or diverging life paths. Sometimes the split is explosive – a build-up of aggravations that leads to anger and recrimination. Sometimes the fissure makes itself clearly visible beforehand – the slow-building crack in the fence that suddenly reaches the point of no return. At other times the split comes out of blue sky for one friend or another. Sometimes the reasons for the split are clear to both parties, sometimes obfuscated to the point of being completely unknowable. The loss of a best friend is wrenching whichever way it happens. It is a source of pain, sadness, yearning, hurt, anger, blame, shame – pick any or all of the above and add a few.

A study of friendships in the United Kingdom surveyed 10,000 people and showed that friendships were ranked as the most important thing in the subjects' lives, even above family. Close friendships provide treasured spaces in which we can be fully ourselves, with all our faults and vulnerabilities. Close friends know and love us as our whole selves, not just as the face or aspect we present to the world. They see the sturdy, resilient, joyous parts of our selves but we also entrust our most fragile and secret selves to the keeping of a close friendship.

Days after Faith's card, I am still finding it hard to believe. It seems impossible that the Faith I know would carry out this ruthless dispatch of a loving friendship. And with the added impossibility that she has refused even the chance to meet and talk it over, it is as if I have been tumbled into some skewed, alternate universe. I weep. More than I have since the first days of Martin's stroke. And for some weeks after, I will find myself having to hold back tears whenever I think of Faith.

I keep expecting to hear from her, even though several weeks have now gone by. Every form of communication – post, telephone, email – becomes touched with the expectation that its next message will be from Faith, that it will be her old familiar voice saying, 'I'm sorry. Let's meet. Let's talk'. But nothing comes.

I think back, trying to understand. Was there something I said? Something I did? Was I needy? Of course I was needy. Anyone going through the continued life-threatening illness of their partner is needy. All close friendships adjust to the different seasons we travel through – one friend is needy at one time, the other at a different time. The balance evens out.

And there is a difference between being needy and being overly demanding in that need. I can understand a friendship wobbling because one friend cannot meet the demands for significantly increased access at a time of crisis. What is one person's reasonable access – a visit once a fortnight – is another person's experience of a choke-hold. But one cup of tea in eight months is nobody's definition of excessive. It cannot have been that. And I am left, as before, mystified.

This is one of the cruelties of unilateral dismissal from a distance. There is no chance to understand. No chance to achieve that wildly overworked term, closure.

When something ends, closure is what we all say we want. As if whatever has ended is an open container that cannot be put away until it has been closed and the contents protected from spillage. And an experience without closure does spill – it leaks all over us as we try to mop it up, sweep it up, push it back into storage where we can label it, file it and understand its nomenclature.

Faith's card has come at a time when Martin is about to discover how precarious the state of his heart is and his epilepsy is as yet uncontrolled. Faith has been on the group email list through which I have been keeping friends posted on the unfolding experience of Martin's health. After receiving Faith's card, I have taken her name off the list. Presumably, if she is insistent on ending the friendship, she does not want contact with me.

It seems the obvious thing to do at the time, but I keep wondering – how can one be deeply and lovingly involved in a friend's life for thirty years and then suddenly not care whether they weather a devastating life crisis or not? I cannot get my head around it. Perhaps Faith really does still care. Perhaps if I offer her a way back in, she will take it.

And so I put her back on the group email list. I feel as if I am opening a back door through which she can re-enter the friendship if she wishes. And when I send the group updates about what is happening with Martin, Faith does reply. A couple of lines – expressing sympathy for what is happening illness-wise, although no mention of what has happened between Faith and me. I am not sure exactly what to make of it, but it seems promising. Perhaps she really does want to keep in contact, to heal the rift.

And then, weeks later, it is my sixtieth birthday. With most of my good friends, birthdays are not an issue – they tend to pass unnoticed. For a few friends, however, marking each other's birthdays with a card or small gift has become a tradition. Faith and I have always put particular thought into each other's birthdays, not just with gifts and cards but through meeting and celebrating each other's special days. There has been a card in the mail from Faith on every one of my last thirty birthdays, and I am fully aware of this as my birthday approaches.

Faith has continued to respond to the group updates. It is beginning to seem as if she does want to remain in touch. And so, on the morning of my sixtieth birthday, I am fully expecting a card. Not our usual celebration meeting and exchange of gifts, but a card on a birthday that is not only a milestone birthday but a birthday celebrated in the midst of extraordinary stress.

And so, when no card comes, the silence is deafening. There is nothing from Faith, no card, no email, no phone message. And that is when I finally, truly understand. It is over. Faith has indeed excised me from her life. Her responses to the group emails were simply expressions of politeness, some show of courtesy that had nothing to do with me or us.

It is shattering once again. And it is a complicated experience. One aspect is the sheer grief of losing a beloved friend who felt like family. It would be painful at any time in any circumstances, but at a time of dealing with ongoing major stresses, it is magnified. And the other extraordinarily distressing aspect is the manner in which the friendship was terminated.

It is so staggeringly unlike the Faith I knew that it brings up the unnerving question of whether I really knew her. And its equally unnerving follow-up – if I didn't know her after such a deep, decades-long friendship, what does that say? And still further along that twisted path – if, on the other hand, I did truly know her, how is it possible that she could have effected such a radical 180-degree turn in her persona and belief system?

I have no answers. And it adds to my fascination with the issues I have been wrestling with since Martin's stroke – the notion of the integrity of self. With Martin, an accident in the brain, the destruction of a group of neurons, has caused a significant shift in his personality – a personality that up till then had been stable for sixty years.

With Faith, something other has caused the shift, but it is no less disconcerting in its implication that our core 'self' may not possess the solid, knowable, reliable existence most of us experience it as having. Who are we if we cannot define ourselves at this level? Is our deepest self simply the product of a particular organisation of brain cells? If they change do we change too at our core level? What circumstances would make us swerve from our most deeply held beliefs and values? And who would we be?

Over the years, Faith has sometimes spontaneously wondered out loud about how she would react if she were a German citizen in Nazi Germany. She has been positive that if she had no dependent family to consider, she would have had no hesitation in putting her life at risk to shelter Jews or other innocents. Her certainty reflects the strength of her belief in this core component of her being – selflessness, compassion and the importance of caring for those in need, even if that caring puts one at risk. I have always admired the courage of people who act altruistically at a time of danger. I would like to think I would have been brave enough to have done the same, but in truth I don't know. Most of us don't know how we would react in such a crisis until it happens. But Faith has always been utterly certain.

It makes her actions in the present even more baffling, but without the opportunity to speak to her, I am limited to my own perspective, which is one-dimensional. And perspective is a key both so elusive and so crucial to understanding, that without it one is lost. I am reminded of an old story…

Three young women die and arrive at the Pearly Gates at the same time. St Peter takes them in for their orientation talk.

'Heaven, as you will see, is a wonderful place', he says. 'Wander around, pick any abode that takes your fantasy. Every possible luxury and lifestyle is available for you. We only have one rule'.

The group nods intently.

'Don't step on a duck', says St Peter. 'That is our only rule and it is enforced firmly'.

No further explanation is forthcoming and the group wanders away, chatting enthusiastically.

So engrossed are they in conversation about the marvels around them that not five minutes have gone by before one young woman feels a sudden and alarming squishiness under her feet followed by an anguished quack. All heads turn. There is a puff of smoke and whoosh, the young woman finds herself handcuffed to a vile, inebriated, foul-mouthed man.

St Peter appears, tut-tutting sadly. 'I'm afraid that's it for eternity', he says. 'Those handcuffs are permanent. You stepped on a duck'.

The two remaining young women are shocked into silence. They pick their way carefully through the streets of heaven. Suddenly, a choir of angels appears. The young women are so transported by the music they forget to look where they are going. And Squish! Quack! One of them has stepped on a duck.

There is the familiar whoosh and, when the smoke clears, the offending young woman finds herself handcuffed to a shambling giant of a man in a prison uniform and with lethally bad breath.

The third young woman is utterly terrified. She puts herself on high alert. No duck within 100 yards is going to get past her search-lit attention. She walks on cautiously and, as time goes by, becomes confident that she now has the hang of it. She has been able to steer clear of anything remotely duck-like. She is just congratulating herself on her sharpened ability when there is a whoosh, a puff of smoke and then the most gorgeous man she has ever seen appears, handcuffed to her.

She is stunned. What has happened?

The gorgeous man, equally startled, looks at her and says 'Damn! I stepped on a duck'.

Like most jokes, this takes as its subject matter the absurdity and tragedy of the human condition. On the one hand, it is a charming and amusing tale about perspective and the illusion of control. It makes us laugh, both heartily and ruefully.

It can also, however, be seen in the light of one of the most common of fairytale themes – the beast marriage.

The fairytale of Beauty and the Beast is deeply familiar to us. A young woman is unwittingly married to a being who is a monster. There have been numerous versions of this folktale, ranging widely over cultures and countries but always with the same theme, an inadvertent partnering with a monster or beast.

The Brothers Grimm version of Beauty and the Beast is the one most of us know. In this version, Beauty's father owes a favour to a fearsome Beast. In return for his life, the father promises to give the Beast his youngest daughter, Beauty, and reluctantly takes her to live with the Beast. Beauty is terrified at first, but the Beast is kind to her. After some time she asks to visit her family at home. Reluctantly, the Beast agrees but only on condition that she return within seven days. Beauty dallies at home, however, and seven days go by. Suddenly, she is woken by a nightmare of the Beast ill and dying. She rushes home to find him deathly ill. Realising that she loves him, she holds him to her heart, tells him so and says that she will marry him. Upon hearing this, the Beast revives and is transformed into a handsome prince. He had been cursed by a witch and was doomed to remain in the form of Beast until the love of a maiden who could accept him as he was reversed the spell.

The Beast husband in these stories is often understood in Jungian terms as representing the Shadow – that part of ourselves we reject and cut off, the part of ourselves we fear, are ashamed of or from which we wish to escape. It is the part of ourselves we try not to know about but that is always there, secretly shackled to us. It takes only stepping on a duck to reveal it.

Most of us try valiantly to avoid these ducks and the shadow selves they may reveal. It is painful to be reminded of our failings – our cowardice, our selfishness, our anger, our greed, the deficiencies in the way we treat others, manage our own lives, or any other of the myriad aspects of self that engender shame, humiliation and the critical judgements meted out by ourselves or others. We box up our shadow selves, deny them, disguise them, hide them and often do a sterling job. But sometimes a duck slips under our feet.

I stepped on my duck at 4.00 am on the morning of 13 June, when I found myself chained to that howling, terrified, alone self, as my computer crashed and all my sense of connection to anyone or anything crashed with it. I cannot un-know that self now. It is a shadow-self that in its insuffiency and dependence frightens me, even horrifies me, and I feel ashamed of it – I should have been bigger, stronger, more self-sufficient. But I also know that it is part of who I am and that I must listen to it and hear what it has to tell me.

Philosophers, of course, have been turning over the questions of who we are and how we judge ourselves and others long before the existence of neuroscientists and psychologists. As part of this quest, some modern philosophers have introduced the concept of moral luck – the notion that circumstances beyond our control affect who we are and how we show ourselves to the world.

In his 1979 essay, Thomas Nagel describes four kinds of moral luck. One of them he calls circumstantial luck. This is the concept that how we behave is determined by the circumstances in which we find ourselves. Moral luck can come in the form of good moral luck, in which circumstances encourage or enable us to show our better selves, or bad moral luck where the reverse happens.

A thought-provoking example of bad moral luck given by Nagel is that of collaborators in Nazi Germany who worked voluntarily in concentration camps and committed reprehensible deeds. If these same people had been living in another country during the war, they would never have had contact with the evils and opportunities of Nazi machinery and might in fact have led very different lives as model citizens. It is the moral luck of finding themselves in Nazi Germany that has opened them up to behaving in abhorrent and morally repugnant ways. In this light, circumstantial moral luck can be seen in some respects as 'duck' theory. If we avoid the ducks, we may have good moral luck. If we step on them, we have bad moral luck and the shadow selves to which we are shackled make a vivid and unsavoury appearance. In the case of Nagel's example, living in Nazi Germany and collaborating represents stepping, if not leaping, on a duck. Living in another country and never being exposed to the Nazi regime and its possibilities, represents avoiding a duck.

On a far more mundane level, Martin's illness was bad moral luck for Faith. If Martin had not been sick, I would not have pressed Faith for that cup of tea. We would have kept in touch by phone and I would simply have assumed that she was busy and not been concerned by the fact that we hadn't got together. I would not have needed the comfort of that cup of tea and a hug. And I would not have had to find out about her shadow side – the ruthlessness, even brutality, she displayed in cutting off our friendship under those circumstances and without explanation or the chance to talk and understand. I would have continued seeing her as the Faith I knew so well – caring, compassionate and altruistic. I would not have had to ask the question of who she really was. And perhaps neither would she. Martin's illness was the duck of bad moral luck that Faith stepped on. What did it change? Who she was at that time? Who she had been? Or who she would be from that time on?

24 February 2010

We are continuing to climb the status ladder of medical personnel at the Prince Edward – yesterday we had our first appointment with a guru of Infectious Diseases. Our series of IDU doctors has gone from registrar to registrar and now to Allan, a very senior consultant.

En route to Infectious Diseases, we accidentally pressed the wrong button on the lift, got out at Respiratory Medicine and were astonished to discover a Prince Edward department we hadn't yet visited.

Allan turned out to be a truly lovely man – warm, experienced and communicative. There were no revelations about the state of Martin's health but a comfort independent of the state of illness comes with being in the hands of a caring, competent doctor.

The highlight of the meeting came when Allan said, 'Would you mind if I give your cardiologist a ring to talk about things?' Martin and I gaped at him. In all of these nine months, he is the first specialist who has expressed a desire to talk to another specialist involved.

And re the question of how long Martin should remain on antibiotics, Allan has come down on the side of taking them for life, as there is no way of knowing whether the bug is dead or dormant and it is too risky to find out.

We are at Carraman Private Hospital today as we see Elizabeth, the neurologist, for a follow-up after Martin's seizure. She looks relieved as she tells us the MRI has shown there was no extra damage from the seizures. She had obviously been worried about that when she ordered the MRI but had masked her worry so well we didn't pick up on it. Her concern was that either the seizures were really strokes or else they were seizures but had caused extra damage. Luckily, it was no to both possibilities, and we are grateful to her calm manner for saving us a few days of extra worry.

17 March 2010

Last week, our two-doctor ration was of a different nature. My regular check-up with my oncologist was on Monday and felt like a tea party – the most enjoyable doctor's appointment I've had for nine months. And for some more light relief we had a dermatologist's appointment for Martin, at which the spot on his toenail turned out to be something as delightfully trivial as a possible fungal infection. And this week, no doctors' appointments at all.

Yesterday, a friend texted me to see how all was going and I texted back, 'It's a week without doctors' appointments. It feels like a holiday!' As I texted this I felt, for almost the first time in nine months, an odd feeling I finally identified as that strangest of experiences – pleasant normality. The Epilim is agreeing with Martin, he is feeling good on it. No doctors' appointments. No crises. I can relax.

And so this morning I am pottering about in the kitchen enjoying that sense of unfamiliar ease when I hear some innocuous-sounding bumping noises and assume Martin is shifting files or drawers. Then odd moaning sounds are added to the mix. I rush upstairs to find Martin having a seizure on bathroom floor. He is unconscious and thrashing wildly.

I rush to the nearest phone, in an adjoining room, to ring Amantha and tell her to phone the ambulance. I don't want to leave Martin alone in the midst of a seizure and in danger of banging his head on the hard tiles.

A few minutes later my landline rings in the next room I scramble to answer it, desperate at having to leave Martin but sure it is the ambulance people. And it is. The ambulance-base secretary is determined to get the history details out of me despite me telling her I am terrified Martin is going to bang his head on the wall or floor and the fact that his moans are loud enough for her to hear on the phone across the corridor in another room.

I keep saying I cannot stay on the phone – that Martin is in another room, that I have to be with him in case he hurts himself, but she is having none of it. She is insisting on bureaucratic details. I am scared that if I get off the phone she will not send the ambulance, but if I don't get off the phone Martin could injure himself.

I rush back and forwards between the phone and Martin. I have put a towel under his head but he is thrashing and jerking crazily. Desperately, I tell her again that I cannot talk – I have to be with him. In response, she actually says, 'Are those his moans I can hear?'

In retrospect, always a sharper form of vision, I should have just told her to shove it and hung up. Instead I keep screaming frantically, 'I can't give you his history now – I have to make sure he doesn't hurt himself', and she keeps saying, 'You have to give me the history for the ambulance call *now!*' with the unspoken threat in her voice 'Or I won't send help'.

Finally, I just slam the phone down and rush to stay with Martin.

After what seems like thirty minutes, but must actually have been less than five, his spasms die down. He is groggy, totally disoriented and having trouble speaking. I sit with him quietly, helping him sit up and wiping off the sweat that has been pouring down his face.

His head is sore where he bumped it in his initial fall but there is no blood anywhere and I just have to hope the bump was a mild one. I am about to collect some towels so he can lie more comfortably on the floor – there is no way I can help him to the carpeted corridor – when there is a ring on the doorbell. The ambulance men have arrived.

Angels were never more welcome. And they *are* angels, wonderful, patient angels. Calm and competent, they check out Martin's vitals, which luckily are okay. They help him down the stairs into a comfortable chair as if he is the only person in the world and they have all the time in the world. They talk about transferring him to the Prince Edward for a fuller examination but I ring his GP and manage to get an appointment later in the day and the ambulance men are happy with that. Only when they are sure everyone is settled do they leave.

The relief of having these superb, steady paramedics checking Martin over is enormous. No more having to second-guess myself about taking him to hospital or not taking him to hospital. No more having to go back and forth in my head asking, 'Is he all right? Is he all right enough? Am I missing something? Do I even know what I'm missing?' The relief of actually having help at a time of such helplessness is profound.

As the professor predicted, Martin has definitely moved on from the partial, simple seizure of his first experience. The last two seizures have been partial, complex seizures, just one rung down from the top of the pole – the grand mal. Martin's seizures are one-sided versions of the grand mal and they are fearsome to watch. Despite my head telling me such a seizure is not fatal, it is impossible to watch without being filled with terror. Everything about it looks so utterly, completely and inhumanly wrong.

Robert, Martin's GP, checks Martin over again and says everything looks fine but he may need a scan because of the worrying bump on his head. It is possible that it caused a slow bleed that is not yet producing neurological signs. He will ring Elizabeth, the neurologist, for her opinion and call us back.

A few hours later, Robert calls back with Elizabeth's thoughts. Although Martin is reaching his acceptable limit of CT scans, Elizabeth thinks this is important enough to warrant one. The MRI will take too long to arrange, so it will have to be a CT. And Martin is to go off the Epilim, which is obviously not working, and start on a new drug, Keppra.

This will be Martin's third anti-epileptic medication. Back in the naive days of his first seizure, when we had been hoping to stay off medication entirely, it had not even occurred to me that if we did need to go onto medication, it might not work.

Dr Google is now sobering me up. I discover the Epilepsy Foundation states that at least fifty per cent of all patients with epilepsy gain complete control of their seizures for substantial periods of time. It goes on to add that another twenty per cent enjoy a significant reduction in the number of seizures. I, of course, am drawn to the fact that this means that for thirty per cent, medication doesn't work. I am staggered by the implications. What does that mean for quality of life? All the ordinary, taken-for-granted freedoms such as driving, swimming and the simple underlying assumption of our everyday lives that our bodies will remain under our conscious control have been swiped from under us.

Still gaping at the thirty per cent possibility that these seizures may become a regular part of our lives, I read on, only to discover that Dr Google has not yet finished with me. There are more shocks in store. The good doctor has found for me a Melbourne University study of more than 1,000 patients with epilepsy. When followed over a number of years, fifty per cent of these people were seizure-free after the first drug regimen tried, thirteen per cent were seizure-free after the second and four per cent were seizure-free after the third. Less than two per cent of the participants stopped having seizures on additional drug treatment courses up to the seventh one tried, and none became seizure-free after that.

These figures simulate for me the experience of being dropped into a bath full of ice cubes. Discounting the Tegretol, which Martin was only on for three days, Epilim was Martin's first proper drug trial. It failed. Keppra will be his second. The Melbourne University study does not engender optimism. I cannot even begin to contemplate this right now, so I put it aside and of course make no mention of it to Martin and Amantha. The Keppra simply has to be effective.

18 March 2010

This morning we see Robert, to pick up the prescription for the 'everything depends on you' Keppra. I instruct Martin not to read the list of side effects, which include depression and are guaranteed to produce depression simply upon reading.

Martin's first question to Robert is, 'Can I take the Keppra last thing at night so it doesn't interfere with my dancing?' Luckily the answer is yes. Robert checks Martin again for any neurological signs indicating bleeding and says it all looks fine but that in the very low likelihood of delayed bleeding into the brain, to watch out for signs of headache and nausea.

'Is there a way of distinguishing the headache/nausea of Keppra side effects from the headache/nausea of brain bleeds?' I ask.

'No', says Robert. 'And that gives me a headache'.

We fill the prescription and head for home. Martin will have to wean himself off the Epilim over the next few days and then we will have another appointment with Robert to oversee the Keppra transfer, an operation that sounds as if it ought to be the sequel to *The Bourne Legacy*.

29 March 2010

Keppra turns out to give Martin a much easier ride than Bourne gave Matt Damon. He is not groggy, dizzy, nauseous, depressed or suffering from any of the other major side effects. He is a fraction more tired than usual but other than that, he is feeling fine. Keppra has passed the side-effects test, now the big question is whether it will pass the effectiveness test. For the answer, we have to wait out the minimum three months.

The unnerving experience of flashbacks continues. At random moments, I glance at Martin seated on the couch, comfortably watching TV and bang, suddenly I see him mid-seizure, thrashing and jerking on the floor, his body gripped in a violent, alien dance. And then – blink – he is back to normal Martin. These images now slap me regularly but unpredictably into a visceral shock.

Worse still is the now constant hyper-alertness I have had to adopt. When Martin is out of sight I am always listening, always alert. I am a deer in a forest of tigers. Every slight sound, every mildest shift of shadow or light clangs alarm. Martin is usually upstairs at his computer and I am downstairs. A hundred times a day I go running up the stairs, adrenaline flushing through my system, alerted by a knock or bumping sound – always careful to slow as I round the corner so that Martin doesn't know I have been racing up the stairs in panic.

Sometimes he has been moving files, sometimes shutting a cupboard door, sometimes doing nothing in particular. I figure my adrenalised state has me imagining sounds, misinterpreting the familiar background track of normality. Eventually I realise that the neighbouring house has a sound tunnel that transports sounds from next door so they seem to be emanating from our house. As the neighbours have two active little boys, many of those sounds not only closely approximate the sounds of someone falling over, yelling or groaning, they are in fact the sounds of someone falling over, yelling and groaning. But run I must, because what if one day those sounds are not coming from a little boy next door but are coming from Martin?

The adrenaline never leaves me. As someone used to being fairly calm, this new constant bath of neurochemicals feels like an unrelentingly tangible presence. If my body were transparent I feel sure I could see the colour of adrenaline as it courses non-stop around and around my system. Every moment, every ordinary, automatic activity is now split by the hyper-alertness that danger could be just a millisecond away. I can no more relax than can a high-speed racing driver taking a curve. Except that for me, the whole of the day and night is a curve; there are no straights in which to stretch out and relax.

On every departure from the house I am dogged by the 'what if...?' What if Martin has a seizure while I am out? What if he falls and hurts himself and no one is there to help? What if the seizure causes more damage to his brain? What if the fall sets off another bleed and there is no one to ring an ambulance?

Each time I walk out the door I triple-check that my phone is with me in case Martin needs help, that I have my keys with me in case Martin has had a seizure and cannot answer the door, that I am not away for too long in case anything happens. The precipice is always an inch away and the cliff is perpetually crumbly. Vigilance is a constant. There is no respite.

At the same time as all my senses are trained on Martin's ongoing safety, I am trying not to let him notice. I don't want him to feel the suffocation and implied danger of constant surveillance. I think wonderingly of the unbelievable pressure on mothers of children with epilepsy. How do they manage the impossible dance between allowing their children a growing independence and the real necessity for constant alertness, not to mention the ongoing fear and anguish the suffering of a child brings? I am in awe of them.

The daily vigilance goes on. As do the neighbouring little boys. The assortment of yells, groans, bumps and cries continues. I race up and down the stairs in a panicked scramble up to a dozen times a day. We buy a small medical alarm Martin can keep near him, but its siren is constantly being set off accidentally, which simply adds to the number of my stair-running alerts.

In the meantime, I am researching the big 'what if…?' What if none of the anti-epileptic medications works? What if Martin is one of the sizeable percentage whose seizures remain impervious to modern medicine? I discover a body of work looking at the impact of diet on epileptic seizures. In particular, some researchers have been evaluating the impact of a diet high in the production of ketones.

The ketonic diet has similarities to the Atkins diet in that it is high-fat and low-carbohydrate. Researchers are unsure as yet of the exact mechanisms by which this helps reduce or prevent seizures, but it seems to have benefited many children for whom medication doesn't work. There are limited studies as well that suggest it might be helpful for adults in this situation.

The diet is draconian and needs the supervision of both a physician and a dietician. Even a single off-diet meal can derail the process. It is a no-cheating, micro-measuring, portion-controlled, no-mistakes-tolerated Maggie Thatcher of a diet. And the possible side effects include kidney stones, high cholesterol and bone fractures.

The side effect I cannot get my head around is the weight-loss aspect. Martin's metabolism is one of the miracles of natural science. No matter how much, how frequently or what he eats, Martin's naturally slim build never gets heavier. In the list of 'I wish I had' when delineating the ideal physical persona, Martin's metabolism ranks well up there with Cate Blanchett's complexion, Elle MacPherson's body and the Pantene girl's hair. Adults use the Atkins diet to lose weight, and the research with children refers to slowed growth or slowed weight gain as a side effect. How could Martin, who has not got an ounce he could afford to lose, follow an Atkins-like diet without becoming skeletal?

In all my reading, I cannot find the answer to that one. I put it aside in the Plan B cupboard, hoping it is one that will never have to be used.

1 April 2010

I am limping around today with a broken toe – the result of a mad rush in the dark to answer a midnight phone call, which turned out to be a wrong number. It is ridiculously frustrating for such an inconsequential injury and will, of course, reduce my running up and down the stairs to the equivalent of a slow-mo action-replay drama.

Not much news from the IDU today, as Martin has not yet had the stress echo, but Allan does say his best guess is that the vegetation on the heart, from the bacteria that caused the endocarditis, is dead vegetation. He then adds casually that the bacteria are easier to kill in the heart than in the brain or spleen. This of course is something we didn't know and no one had mentioned.

There are several gulps as we assimilate this new information. All my concerns had focused on whether the bacteria in Martin's heart were dead. I had completely forgotten that scans also showed some in his spleen and that of course the bacteria that had broken off and headed for his brain were still in there. All we can do, however, is hope and enact that easy-to-say and hard-to-endure phrase 'watch and wait'.

Throughout this whole wild ride, Martin's ability to go with the flow has been extraordinary. He has put up stoically with horrifying conditions, with disability, with the slog of continued day-after-day rehab work and at times small gains. When I tell him I admire his ability to just get on with it, he shrugs and says that he doesn't worry, he just rolls with the punches. And I am suddenly struck by what a brilliant team we have made.

I am not good at rolling with the punches. I try to change the punches or figure out how to shift the game. And that is indeed what I have been doing. I have been researching, finding doctors, making phone calls, always thinking two steps ahead. That has been my role. And it has been made so much easier for me by

Martin being willing to get his head down, tolerate the abysmal conditions and steadily do the rehabilitation work that needs to be done on a daily basis. He has not needed to research or plan ahead – I am doing that. And I have not needed to keep motivating him to action – he is taking care of that. If he hadn't been, I would not have been able to do my job so well. And if I hadn't been doing my job, he would not have made anywhere near the recovery he has now attained. We have been the perfect team.

And I suddenly realise, too, that this response to a life-threatening health crisis – a day-by-day 'roll with the punches' approach – was what Martin also took during my two experiences with ovarian cancer. Then, I was the patient too ill to take on the relevant research tasks, and I think back now and realise that Martin, the computer analyst, didn't ever open up his computer to research ovarian cancer or its treatment. I hadn't thought about it at the time but I now realise how strange that seems. We both knew I was facing a possible death sentence but Martin's response was to put a lid on it – the possibility of my death was too overwhelming for him to face. My response is to open the box. Each of us expresses a particular way of coping with anxiety. Each strategy has its pros and its cons. And in a wonderful confluence of circumstances, we have each been able to bring to this crisis our best strengths.

29 April 2010

It is finally time for Martin's stress echocardiogram. Peter the cardiologist meets us afterwards to tell us the results. The stress echo shows borderline–severe regurgitation, which means the surgery should be scheduled sooner rather than later and we should make an appointment with him in July and go forward from there. 'Go forward' being the terminology for picking surgeons and scheduling operation dates. Suddenly the spectre of open-heart surgery on a heart with a probably dead, possibly dormant, bacterial infection seems terrifyingly real.

We calculate that any date later than October is not good, as we don't want Martin's post-surgery recuperation weeks to overlap with doctors' post-surgery recuperation weeks of the Christmas holidays. And if we can go through till July with no seizures, we can feel confident that the Keppra is indeed working to control Martin's epilepsy, an important factor in the scheduling of surgery. So we are hoping for some time between July and October. The next step is to find a cardiac surgeon and get their opinion.

In this we are helped by two friends, who have gone ahead and done the practical research for us. The name on both of their lips is that of George. He has operated on both of them and they sing his praises. Robert, Martin's GP, adds to the praise when we mention George's name, and Peter the cardiologist says when we ask him, 'If anyone can repair Martin's mitral valve, it would be George'.

I have had a bug for the last couple of weeks and, ironically, after surviving the conditions and contagions of South-Central Rehab without so much as a hint of a cold, Martin has now caught one in the comforts of home. So far it is just a very sore throat and no temperature but I am on the alert, as high temperature can cause a seizure. However, it is eight weeks and three days since his last seizure so we are daring to feel optimistic. In a few weeks we see Elizabeth the neurologist, and if Martin has had no seizure by then she will let him drive. Hard to imagine the relief we will feel to think that the seizures are under control, although I suspect my thigh muscles will immediately begin to deteriorate as the need to charge up and down the stairs in response to the bumping sound of a bird landing on the roof abates.

26 May 2010

I am re-reading my old updates today – I stopped sending them out on a daily basis a few months ago. There I was back then, talking as if one month was a vast amount of time and here I am nearly twelve months down the track with more hurdles still to come. It is astounding to think that so much time has passed since that first plunge into crisis. And that there has been no respite since. With horrifying predictability, as each crisis begins to feel familiar and in some ways manageable, a new one erupts.

My toe is at last beginning to recover from the after-effects of the midnight phone call, although my foot and leg are still painful. They are just starting to get better as the weather is starting to get worse, so the four days of sunshine and walking that I envisaged for the Easter holidays have disappeared. It is a small thing but it has hit me too hard. I constantly forget what a tightrope I am walking on. My mood, normally stable and resilient, is now easily tipped over – 'labile' is the word for it.

The root of the word 'labile' comes from *labi* – meaning to fall or to slip – and it feels remarkably appropriate. The drop in mood these days when I am overtired or overstressed is like a fall, followed by the beetle-on-its-back experience, without the energy to do the wriggling around necessary to right myself. Eventually I do find the energy, but what is most frightening about the experience is the sense of being completely drained, of having no energy at all, not even a skerrick in reserve.

And there is also the aloneness of being so fatigued that even breathing can feel like an effort, and I am too tired to pick up the phone and ring friends despite the fact that I would welcome talking to them. This exhausted sense of isolation is intensified by the reality that this long into Martin's illness, people don't phone or email regularly to see how things are going in the way they did during the first few weeks. They assume things are stable, that there is no immediate crisis. And it is true, there *is* no immediate life-threatening crisis as there was in the early days of Martin's stroke. The crises, however, have been ongoing, major and deeply stressful, although without the drama of those first few days. And the phone calls and expressions of caring are needed just as much in the weeks and months of grinding, ongoing tension as they are in the initial days.

The epilepsy has been more debilitating for both of us than I could possibly have imagined. Every minute of every day, I have had to be on high alert – a hyper-vigilance that has been constant, necessary and utterly exhausting.

When a friend does ring, it is immediately nourishing and renewing. The sense of being cared about is restorative and a friend's voice, even without their physical presence, is the most warming vehicle for that message. When I read a study showing that interstate college students' levels of cortisol (a stress hormone) dropped when they talked to their mothers on the phone and not just in person, I am not surprised. The voice does things that text cannot replicate.

I am lucky in that I have dear and loving friends – I am in no doubt about this. In normal times, however, with busy working lives, we might go for weeks without being in contact. And in normal times this has never been a problem. I know they love me, that it is mutual and that we are there for each other.

On the introvert–extrovert continuum, I tend towards the introversion side. I relish spending time with my good friends but I also need time to myself, I prefer one-on-one time to group lunches. I would rather read than gossip. I like talking with friends; I don't like parties. Sometimes I have less of this than I want, sometimes plenty – the balance evens out. What I am struck by now, however, is the vulnerability of being in the position where I need more people-contact than I usually do.

The loss of Faith has played a large part in this as well. Out of my close friends, Faith had been the one with whom I spoke most regularly and frequently. Her absence has left a painful hole in my life that has not been filled. And so, at a time when I need more talk, more contact with friends, I have significantly less than I had, say, a year ago.

I feel it acutely – my fantasies revolve around my friends being retired and at leisure, living around the corner. I ration myself, putting them on a mental roster so as not to put too great a burden on any one time-pressed friend.

I work in a solo psychology practice, without the daily or regular conversational contact with colleagues that a work setting often provides. I notice that if I have one long chat with a friend once a week, I am fine. If I go for two weeks without that kind of contact, my mood drops. I am fascinated by the predictability of this.

A 2010 Arizona study looked at the differing impacts of pleasant small talk versus meaningful conversation. Somewhat to the researchers' surprise, the results suggested that people who had regular deep and meaningful conversation, even about difficult topics, felt significantly happier than those who had a higher proportion of pleasant chitchat. The researcher concluded that the notion that 'as long as you surf on the shallow level of life you're happy, and if you go into the existential depths you'll be unhappy' didn't hold.

In fact, conversations about meaningful topics, even distressing ones, leave us happier for two essential reasons: as humans, we have a need to find and create meaning, and we are also hardwired to be social animals who need connection with others. Meaningful conversations speak to both of those drives and needs. It is through discussing issues, particularly difficult or emotional issues, that we are able to create a meaningful narrative around them. At the same time, we are bonding with the person with whom we are talking – connecting with them at a level that allows us a sense of knowing and being known by them.

Years later, I am having a conversation with a friend I have not seen for years. She, too, has been through some very traumatic years, and talks of how she needed friendship and talking more than usual during that time and took care to ration her contact with friends, so as not to overload any one friendship. I nod instantly in the been-there-done-that gesture of recognition.

Throughout this time, I have been continuing intermittently with that other kind of 'talking' via my regular email updates to friends. But I have thought to myself that I should also write about this in a different way, exploring it as I did with my memoir *Eating the Underworld*. That writing was both a literary journey through life-threatening illness and a discovery of self, a way of creating something of meaning and value from difficult experience. It was paradoxically both stressful to revisit many of those experiences and yet at the same time deeply nourishing to discover the narrative within them. In addition to the transformative power of words and story, it is as if the act of creation itself in some way acts as a counterbalance to the decimation of sorrow and loss.

People who have read the updates are also urging me to write about this, to expand the updates into a book. But although I make half-hearted attempts to sit down at the computer, I don't write. I am too tired, too busy, too fraught, with as many reasons for not writing as to write. But the real reason, the invisible reason, which I only begin to discover gradually, is that I don't know the ending of this story.

None of us, of course, ever knows the ultimate ending to our story, but experience is episodic – we live chapters in our lives, we have the concept of journeys, where there is a goal, a destination, an end point. And a journey is just another name for a story – our story – with its beginning, its middle and its end. And that is where the memoirist generally starts – regardless of what the written words say in those first pages – at the end, rather than the beginning, because a memoir details a chapter in a life and a chapter implies a start and a finish, an overall view. You already know what has happened when you begin. And the beginning of a journey is understood through the filter of its finish.

Writing this beginning without knowing the ending feels frightening. I am terrified of the ending. I feel a superstitious fear that writing down the words will set something in motion. Perhaps some fate that has forgotten about us will have its memory jogged by the metaphorical sound of tapping keys, crawl out of its cave and deliver whatever horror those final paragraphs contain. I don't want to wake it. And so I prevaricate, evade and delay.

In the end it is the dark that sends me to the keyboard. We are entering winter and the last time winter began, a year ago, was the week Martin had his stroke. Each day I left the house in the damp, cloud-heavy mornings to spend the day by Martin's hospital bed. By the time I left each evening, darkness had lowered itself and I would arrive back to a silent, unlit house. My first act on entering was to turn on all the lights – a response to something far more primitive than the knowledge of greenhouse gases and ecologically sound living. Even today, when Martin has been home for months, if he leaves the light on in his room, I cannot bring myself to turn it off. Some deep and archaic superstition has equated light with life, and although I can happily turn off the light in every other room, I cannot bring myself to enact the harmless gesture of clicking off the light switch Martin has carelessly left on in his room in daylight.

Autumn was blue-skied and sunny but winter has come with the suddenness of a shutter dropping, with the sky turned to thickened shadow and the air suckingly chill. The morning light is barely light at all and it is this visceral experience of darkness that has driven me back to writing. It is a deep, instinctive response to the primal need for stories – those age-old charms shared around fires in the frightening lightlessness of night, their task to ward off and name the dark when there was no other way to do so.

This winter is the coldest Melbourne has had for years. In the streets and shops people are rubbing their hands, emitting the loud 'brrs' of exaggerated shivering and complaining about the cold. I am wearing two jumpers and a knitted ear-warming headband but still I can feel the cold. Inside me, as if the number of outer layers is meaningless, immaterial, I feel cold. It is as if my body has subterranean memories of always walking through winter to get to Martin in hospital. For the first time in more than thirty years I get chilblains on my toes. I have to cover my ears at night or else, in a centrally heated house, the painful cold of my ears will wake me. Each night, I wrap a bandanna around my head, with the ends hanging down as flaps to cover my ears, and head for bed in Florence of Arabia style.

Cold, I am discovering, has an emotional temperature as well as a Centigrade one. We have always known this, of course – our everyday language tells us so: our blood runs cold with terror, we have chills of dread, we shiver with fear. I have reacted to weather before – who has not felt uplifted by blue skies and sunshine and dimmed by leaden skies? – but never like this. It is as if there is no insulating layer between me and the cold. As if the cold is taking over not just my body, but my self, the person I think of as 'I'.

In books and films, winter weather and storms are the backdrop to doom and tragedy. You know that when the story begins, either verbally or visually with 'It was a dark and stormy night', someone is in trouble. People are lost in winter, killed, threatened, frozen, injured. It is the winter of Narnia where the witch's curse means it is always winter and Christmas never comes.

But in some stories, something else happens. Winter is also the season of magical storms. In Shakespeare's *The Tempest* it is the storm, terrible though it is, that brings what is needed to Prospero on his isolated island. The storm is the energy of winter that forces us to action, whether it is the action of running to safety, securing shelter or stoking the fire. And so, with the computer as my campfire, I finally sit down and begin to write. To take myself back to the beginning before catching up to the known present and the unknown future.

The Neighbouring Bed in the Neurology Ward

1

They are the opposite of fog
in a room where light is not the answer
and anyway, has nothing to say
to the face of the young man
who's a traveller
in the bed on the platform
of ward 43. They are doing all
that is untaught
to a sister, two mothers
in the space between clocks
between curtains in the closed
heart of the ward-room,
they have stored up hope
like all the rocking ships
of the desert,
but this is a different terrain
where nothing is left
but to call through deep water and pray
that their voices will turn him towards them.

2

The neighbouring bed is what you see
in between watching
the breath shift in and out of your husband's body.
His face, astonishingly still
imprinted in the image of himself
being himself, but only in sleep,
the other land of the living.
There was a flood this morning
in the delicate unskinned shell –
the brilliant mollusc of living
that wrinkles under the skull.
The levees went down

and all of the inhabitants subsided
into silence.
The words drowned.

3

An hour ago he was awake and seeking
them – words, those skiddy fish
of the self, schooled in between
seeing. He is looking, you can see
he is looking, for nets, for bait,
for the slippery hooks of our need
to be in the world in particular clothing.
He is trying, you can see he is trying,
for what we haul in each day
without thinking: the slithering masses
of sound that are our names for this, for that,
for everything that matters.

4

To get to this ward
you must pass a river.
Sunlight only makes it hungrier
to gobble your reflection.
Stride by stride
the shaking part of you
bobbles through it, always remembering
never to look behind.
From the hospital room, I imagine
the water, a miles-off murmur
of words, of something faintly querulous
and urgent
telling me to understand
there is always a river to cross,
someone to fight for,
something to lose

again and again
that you are never allowed to find
in the same way twice.

5

Lifetimes ago, between the gold and marooned pages
of Arthur Mees' *Children's Encyclopaedia,*
I lived like an island reading
the sea – the waves' braille
gulled and ancient, teaching me what to see:
Be careful of ravens,
particularly those with a penchant
for older men's shoulders.
Watch out for swans that seem too confident.
And when encountering curses
choose your leaves first –
opposition has a way of turning
into vegetation.
That was where I first found them –
Baucis and Philemon
those two elder Greeks who knew
the laws of hospitality
and what to do with the knock on your door
and the strangers breathing
with odd unfamiliarity.

6

They came as a test
of course. And those who beware
the uninvited know they tend to travel
in pairs. Zeus – the brother
who made the killing, head gunslinger
of heaven and earth. And Hermes, governor
of truth and lies, merchants and herds, thieves,
stars, guests, runners and eloquent speech:

So many things to do, there was nothing to do
but pronounce him god over boundaries,
the interstitial and whatever steps out of spaces
to become itself. Or the other.
Rejected by every house but this they step in, invited,
accept scarce food, a fire, drink. Their generous hosts are somewhat
puzzled when the lone, thin goose runs
to the stranger begging his protection.

7
Radiance revealed, they drop on shivered knees
and hear the impossible
golden voice proclaim that they can have anything.
Only to serve, is their wish, they say. Politic
or genuine? It doesn't matter. Have more, the gods urge.
A shy glance. 'May we die in the same instant,
entwined with each other?' The gods nod yes and disappear
to destroy the rest of the neighbourhood – a flood
of course. They lived for years before simultaneously
turning into trees.
And at the age of eight, when you have not yet
swallowed the moment
of fruit and the ledge
seems knowable and you are an acrobat,
that was the wish I could not understand.
Back then.

8
By the bed on the right,
someone's released the blind
and the wall flicks open a surprised
eyelid. How far up we are
above the street, which is small
but authentically created –
long, cross-loops of cars unravelling,

the angled, open mouths
of permanently surprised umbrellas,
their travellers waiting to step down-
stage from the pavement's strict edges
where the men from Brink's
stitch down their final security details
and roll off, leaving space
traced with the skitter of recent
rain-work. From a doorway,
one lone man emerges
to observe the shining sleet of absence.

9
Meanwhile, the winter light
leaks through the windows, reminding
us of what it isn't
or perhaps trying to tell us
what it is. How much further it had to come
than easy summer, where the earth positions
itself like a cat, lapping it up in the shortest possible
way. How it came through the cold hole of space,
how it came even though the sun turned away,
or was it the earth to which it was offering itself?
How it came anyway, withered and weak, ashamed
of its skinny bony self, so much less
than the other sun was offering.
How we turned it away, or was it ourselves
we turned? How it knew it was not
what we wanted, not even what we had earned
but it was all that we had.
So it came anyway.

Part 3

17 June 2010

I have only just stopped having flashbacks of Martin in the throes of a seizure. The flashbacks had been happening several times a week – so freezingly gripping that even though their actual period of existence was only a few seconds, they had a half-life of hours.

In the last two weeks, though, I have noticed, with the oddness of waking from a dream, that as I walk, talk and do everyday things with Martin, it feels normal. As if somehow I have returned from the terrifying scrabble for life in the wilderness to the comfort and stability of the suburbs.

One of the dictionary definitions of normality is 'conforming to a regular pattern'. Normality is reliable. Days may vary but their core aspects stay steady – the stability of the space you live in, your role, your identity, your family, your friends. Normality is the opposite of disruption, the opponent of shifts, shocks and losses.

It is both comforting and frightening to feel myself relaxing into the arms of normality. Comforting because it feels so good. Frightening because I know that this normality is only the thinnest of shells. But when I am in it, I cannot remember the old feelings of impending doom, of rending, horrifying loss. I can remember that I had those feelings, but I cannot recapture them. It is like a wound that has healed over – you can see the scar, you can know what was there and what it felt like, but you cannot feel it.

It is fascinating to see how my mind fades the intensity of the feelings of dread, sorrow and loss that were so much a part of the last year. It is as if as soon as there is a break in the weather – patches of sun and only scattered showers instead of rain – the mind takes its own holiday, puts coverings over the furniture of grief and heads outside to pretend it is normal. With the cardiologist's appointment on Friday, things may rapidly shift to a different scene, but for the moment, I feel stressed, exhausted but otherwise myself.

I am in fact so exhausted that I have regularly been doing things like putting my shoes in the dirty laundry basket and socks in the freezer, but as I look over the past year, I can see that although we have been unlucky, we have also been lucky. The stroke didn't kill Martin or permanently disable him; he has made an excellent recovery. The endocarditis was diagnosed before it could cause another stroke or heart attack and has responded to treatment. The third anti-epileptic drug, Keppra, is working and Martin is feeling good on it. These are all pieces of good luck, just as the things that necessitated them were bad luck.

And in another piece of good luck, this morning Elizabeth the neurologist gives Martin the thumbs up to drive. It is three months since he has had a seizure, and it looks as if the Keppra has come through on the third-time-lucky principle. It is a staggering relief to feel that the seizures are under control and that my constant state of over-alertness can begin to truly abate.

2 July 2010

This afternoon we see Peter the cardiologist to organise another stress echogram for Martin. Peter asks how Martin is doing with activities and blanches a little when Martin tells him his heartbeat regularly gets up to 140 during folk dancing. Peter suggests trying not to go beyond 120.

'Impossible', Martin snorts to me as we walk to the car park. 'A heart beat of 140 while dancing couldn't possibly be a problem'.

Next dance session, with a proactive blaze of initiative, Martin wears a heart rate monitor while dancing. He drops off the resulting graphs to Peter with a note asking whether he should still stick to Peter's edict about not going above a heart rate of 120 while dancing. Peter, obviously dazzled by this presentation of pre-, during and post-dance heart-rate graphs, rewards Martin with a phone call saying he is now allowed to dance without having to stick to 120.

And Peter also says that in view of the latest stress echo results, we should now start the process of consulting George, the cardiac surgeon, to make a date for surgery. He adds that Martin's situation is trickier than the average cardiac patient's and that the particular chorda that has torn is considered a more difficult one to repair, but the surgery is necessary, so it will be fingers-crossed time again. We have an appointment with George on Wednesday in his rooms at the Royal Melbourne Hospital.

28 July 2010

The journey to George's rooms brings with it a moment of insight unrelated to cardiology. As we finally emerge from the car, I realise there was a good reason for the location of the old psychiatric facility at nearby Royal Park – it was built to accommodate all the Royal Melbourne Hospital patients who had gone insane while attempting to locate a parking space within a ten-kilometre radius of the RMH.

Forty minutes of circling the RMH vicinity had still netted us no discernible parking space. We had finally been driven to park in a one-hour metered spot – the only one we could find within a half-day's trekking distance – figuring that we would just have to wear the over-time parking fine if an inspector happened by. And included in the reckoning is the fact that a parking fine would be cheaper than several days' stay as an inpatient at the local psychiatric unit.

George is terrific – warm, expert, an excellent communicator. He spends a full hour with us, explaining everything, including the increased risks to which Martin's stroke and endocarditis have left him susceptible with this surgery. After detailing all this he pauses, however, and then says he thinks he has a good chance of repairing, rather than replacing, Martin's mitral valve.

The effect of these words is instant and unnervingly visceral – as if several suitcases of lead have suddenly been vaporised from my shoulders. For seconds, I feel disorientingly, giddyingly light. With a successful repair, there would be no concrete block hovering inches above our heads for the first time in sixteen months. It is unimaginable to contemplate. Later, after coming home from George's appointment, I will discover that I am so physically exhausted I can barely climb the stairs, as if my muscles have drained themselves by holding up all that weight and are now utterly spent.

George shows us the artificial metal valve that would be needed if a repair were not possible – a circular little gadget with flaps that click as they work. He flaps it around to demonstrate and the effect is much like one of those party noisemakers. George explains again the negatives for Martin associated with having a metal replacement – his increased risk of infection, the need for lifelong blood thinners and then, the kicker, the new role of ambulant party noisemaker. This comes in particularly handy for pirate-themed fancy-dress parties. Less handy when sitting next to paranoid passengers on aeroplanes. Hopefully, however, Martin will be required to purchase any future noisemakers, like the rest of us, from the appropriate shops.

Martin has to have an angiogram, to check his arteries are okay – no reason to suppose that they are not – and then we will be able to set the actual date. With a choice of the RMH and the Lawson hospital, we have chosen the Lawson. There are a few reasons for this – parking and sanity being at the top of the list.

12 August 2010

My deep fatigue is a constant companion. It will lift temporarily and then plummet down to cloak me again. And each time that happens, I think with surprise, 'Why am I so tired?' And it takes me a few seconds to remember that I have had no respite from serious life-threatening crises for more than a year.

While chatting to a friend, I mention that it has been fourteen months now of constant medical crises and she says with surprise, 'Yes, that's right, I keep forgetting'. It is extraordinarily odd to me that I too keep forgetting. I feel as if I am split into various selves in a way that is far more pronounced than I have ever experienced.

There is the public self, doing the things I normally do – chatting to people, getting things done with my usual fairly cheerful persona; my professional self – teaching, supervising, seeing patients; my at-home self, more tired and rather obsessively absorbed in creating things – fabric art, restyled op-shop garments; my interior self – engrossed in sorting through experiences, feeling, thinking, wondering; and then the devastated self I see much less of now. She arrives just occasionally when I am particularly exhausted, in the grip of especially intense fatigue.

She, my devastated self, was there much more frequently in the earlier months after the stroke. Her appearance is now so infrequent that I feel startled when she pops up. And yet, I am superstitious enough, scared enough of her, to fear that just by writing this I am tempting Fate to step up her appearance rate.

There are two images I have of this devastated self. One is captured in the moment I howled like a dog, sitting at my desk in the dark early hours of the morning, unable to sleep and with my computer suddenly broken, cut off, it seemed, from every living being on the planet.

The other image is that of total depletion – a sucked-dry exhaustion where breathing and the other associated biomechanics of life seem to take effort. The feeling is frightening, as if my self – that energy I think of as 'me' – is being leached away. What is left feels too fine – pin-thin and brittle – as if the very structure of my self is losing the ability to support me. And paradoxically, at the same time as I feel light enough to be substance-less, I also feel too inertly heavy to move.

Sometimes in this state I have just enough energy to read. If I can open the right book I may be able to disappear into it for a while and emerge nourished. I have ready-to-read books stacked in a pile by my bed. My taste is eclectic. I am reading memoirs, literary fiction, humorous detective stories, works of fantasy. There are only two criteria as far as I can tell for what allows me to enter the book. It must be well written so that I can be nourished by the beauty or wit of the language, and it must contain someone

I want to spend time with. This lack of energy is acting as the most discerning gate-barring literary critic – it will not allow me entrance to a place where there is no sustenance.

The extreme fatigue usually stays for a few days and then gradually settles back to my new norm of significant fatigue. During those days of particularly intense fatigue, my mood drops too, as if energy is akin to light and its absence leaves only a dulled twilight. When I first noticed this conjunction of fatigue and mood, I was unsure which was cart and which was horse. Now, unless there is a crisis related to Martin's health precipitating my mood, it feels clear that the physical fatigue is the horse and my emotional descent is the hoof-following cart. And when the fatigue has passed and I am back to normal, or whatever passes for normal in this extraordinary time; it is hard to recall the country of flat, hopeless exhaustion I have just passed through.

30 August 2010

Yesterday, Peter's office rang to give Martin the date of his angiogram and to tell him it would be an overnight stay. I had for some reason expected it to be a day procedure, and the simple, unexpected event of discovering I will be leaving Martin in hospital overnight once more unpredictably and immediately turfed me into reliving the two months of leaving Martin in hospital, and the old feelings of fear and desolation.

I am constantly stunned to remember that far more devastating losses are being experienced every minute of every day by multitudes of people who are all around me. The faces we pass without seeing, the people we do transient business with, the nodding acquaintances, all carrying their losses and stories hidden from our view, moving unnoticed through our ordinary streets.

5 September 2010

The angiogram experience yesterday started with a winning attempt by Carraman as it tried for its place in the 'how insane can we make them?' hospital race. We arrived on time, did all the necessary paperwork and were told to sit over there until we were summoned. We sat. We sat some more. We sat some more still. Then Martin's phone rang. It was Carraman, indignantly asking us where we were. We were in Carraman, we said.

As the nurse walked us down to the ward, she regaled us with tales of how unreliable the lifts were and how just yesterday she had found herself alone in the lift, stuck between floors, unable to open the doors or summon help and panicking.

'Where are the stairs?' I asked nervously.

After that start, however, Carraman improved its game considerably and we were impressed by its pleasantness and efficiency.

Today, the results are through and Peter pronounces Martin's arteries to be in excellent condition, although the angiogram did confirm the previous findings that his mitral valve is leaking severely and that surgery is in order sooner rather than later. As Peter reported to me on the tiptop shape of Martin's arteries, he said, 'That's what healthy living does for you'.

'And folk dancing', I added.

On arriving home, we ring George the surgeon's rooms and we now have an actual date for Martin's mitral valve surgery – it will be on 1 October. It has been lurking on the indeterminate horizon for so long that it is unnerving to think it is all going to be happening in only four weeks.

'Cliff-face living' is the phrase that keeps running through my mind. It is as if for the last fifteen months I have been hauling myself up a cliff face by notches, crevices and cracks – hands and toes struggling to find a grip – and regularly being stunned when a piece of the cliff breaks off and falls away. Finally, three-quarters of the way up, I have found a niche. A large one – cave-sized – in which I can haul myself up and rest. This is where I have been for the last three weeks, in a place that is both safe and unsafe. I know that at some point I will have to venture out again, scrambling for the handholds, praying that my fingers and toes can follow the notches to push upwards, slowly upwards, until at last my hands feel the longed-for contours of the top and I can lever myself up and slowly roll over onto flat, safe land.

19 September 2010

I feel caught in a peculiar stasis, which is also paradoxically full of movement as the days and then weeks pass. I am in the back of a car on a journey to an unknown but dangerous destination. I am not in the driver's seat. Not even in the front passenger seat. I am that most impotent of car inhabitants – the back-seat driver – worried, scared, trying to make a difference and utterly powerless.

When we met with George, the cardiac surgeon, a couple of months ago, he mentioned that Martin was a good candidate for a new technique involving an incision in the side of his ribs, as opposed to the traditional method, which involves coming in from the front and breaking and spreading the rib cage. George said the side incision had the advantage of not involving broken ribs and thus a faster healing time. He had performed thirty of the side techniques as opposed to hundreds of the traditional technique. He left it to us to choose which we would prefer.

After our initial burst of enthusiasm about the shorter healing process, I start to obsess about the number thirty and whether thirty procedures means you are still on a learning curve or alternatively that you could do it in your sleep.

I have a chat to a surgeon friend who has mastered any number of surgical techniques and who sensibly says there is no answer to that question – it is different for every surgeon and every procedure. So when George rings to ask what we have decided about the surgical alternatives he had offered, I ask if we can schedule another appointment with him to talk some more about it. He says of course and we organise a time in the coming week.

I spend the next few days wondering if I am being obsessive, neurotic, nitpicking – and various other unflattering adjectives– in taking so much time to make up my mind about which technique would be best. It is so tempting to pick the technique with the faster recovery but I keep feeling there is a question I need to ask, that something I don't know needs to be factored in. Finally, I give up obsessing about whether I am being obsessive and sit down to prepare the usual list of questions, knowing that 'the' question is not on it.

22 September 2010

Our appointment with George is this morning. We head out early in order to factor in the extra forty-five minutes required to seek out a parking spot. Camping overnight would be the better game plan, but finally we achieve success and head to George's waiting room. Three minutes before George calls us in, I suddenly realise what the missing question is.

'What technique will give you the best conditions for a repair as opposed to a replacement?' I ask.

And as soon as I say it, just as in all those fairytales about asking the right question, solving the riddle, picking the right name, the answer comes clearly. Going in from the front of the chest provides greater access and makes it easier for the surgeon, George says. While the frontal, rib-breaking technique is rougher on the body and has a longer recovery time, it has the advantage of offering more working space for the surgeon to apply his various mending techniques and therefore offers the better chance of a successful repair versus a replacement.

Decision made.

George is continuing to impress us – as well as his superb reputation as a surgeon, he is warm and engaged, and we feel very comfortable with him. He will organise a neurologist to oversee the extra anti-epileptic meds Martin will need during surgery, and an infectious diseases consultant to check out the endocarditis aspects, so Martin will have his own entourage of specialist medicos while at the Lawson.

30 September 2010

Martin is to be admitted to the Lawson this morning in preparation for his surgery tomorrow. Martin, Amantha and I set out for the

Lawson at 11.30 am, knowing that the next time we are all in the car together our lives will have been changed.

In the one brief interval during the day that I am out of Martin's sight – finding something to eat at the cafeteria that doesn't look as if it has been soaked in oil, rolled in lard and then triple-fried – the anaesthetist drops by and then ten minutes after I leave for home, George the surgeon comes by – so my timing is reliably out of kilter. Martin has long chats with both of them, however, and they are looking after him well.

Part of the 'day before surgery' options available at the Lawson is a tour of the Intensive Care Unit (ICU), where open-heart surgery patients will spend time immediately following their surgeries. There is a regular tour at 4.00 pm. You wait to be collected by your tour guide, in what feels unnervingly like a dystopian version of Disneyland. There are five of us – a young woman and her father as well as Amantha, Martin and me. We swap medical details while waiting and are chatting about surgeons when a young woman arrives. We stand obediently and are led off for our tour. As we are about to get into a lift, a trolley, complete with patient, appears, being wheeled along the corridor. This is obviously the equivalent of Mickey Mouse making a personal appearance at the Disney Worlds, and we are all invited to gather around the trolley's inhabitant and observe. Luckily, the patient is unconscious and unaware of his role in the tour.

We are then gathered together for a peek into the ICU, a place that reminds me of the underground fortresses staffed by villains in superhero movies – sinister places filled with a multitude of beeping machines and uniformed worker-attendants.

The occupant of each ICU bed is attached to a mass of machinery and tubing and is either unconscious or in deep, frozen sleep. The nurses glide around with sober expressions, tending to the sleepers or, more accurately, to their machines. It is one of the grimmest rooms I have ever looked in on.

It is a relief to get back to Martin's room, which is airy, light and large. His surgery is scheduled for 1.30 pm tomorrow and, if all goes well, should take about four hours. George has said he will either phone me or come by and talk to me after the surgery. Amantha and I plan to get to the hospital at about 9.30 am tomorrow so we can be with Martin for the morning.

In the lead-up to his surgery, I have made a hypnosis tape for Martin. There is evidence that hypnosis aids recovery from surgery. It is helpful at many levels – it tends to speed up recovery time, the patient requires less anaesthetic, it assists in pain control, reduces anxiety and generally smooths the post-surgical recovery path. In order to make Martin's hypnosis tape, I have had to research thoroughly all the things that can go wrong in open-heart surgery. It has been a sobering experience. Apart from the fact that it is major and invasive surgery, particular aspects of the procedure carry their own unique dangers. Chief among these is that for a period of time, the patient's heart is stopped and maintenance of the essential aspects of life, such as the flow of oxygen to the brain, is taken over by a machine outside the body. The chilled body temperature that is also standard for these surgeries is another special factor.

One of the problems that can arise in addition to the normal surgical risks is the passage of tiny air bubbles through the heart–lung machine, which doesn't filter as finely as the human heart and lungs. The chilled temperature can also prove a hurdle for the body to overcome as normal temperature is restored. And tiny mini-strokes, caused by the air bubbles, are possible. Some specialists think they are likely to be the cause of the often-reported fogginess, temporary personality changes or mild, temporary cognitive impairment some patients experience post-operatively. And depression is also very common after open-heart surgery. It is useful to be aware of this, as the spouses and carers of many patients have been shocked and frightened by the appearance of these symptoms, not realising they are temporary and common. Depression, of course, whenever it appears, is something that should be attended to with professional help.

1 October 2010

On the morning of his surgery, Martin has been playing his tape and is in good spirits. Close to the appointed time, the orderly comes to wheel Martin down to the surgical suite and tells Amantha and me we are welcome to come along. We enthusiastically follow. We are ushered through the doors of the surgical suites to a large bare room that resembles the deserted stands of airline check-in counters when the plane has departed and the next is not due till tomorrow. Martin's is the only trolley in the large unfurnished space, Nurses move through every now and then with the uncanny silence of slippered feet, but otherwise there is no sign of life or activity. Welcome to the holding room.

I have been used to farewelling surgical patients at the sliding doors of the surgical suites, so this is a new one for me. The holding room, it seems, is the anteroom to the surgical theatres, where the patients are kept until the surgeon is ready for them. Martin is lying on his trolley wrapped in blankets but fully conscious. The nurse who checked him in has left and we are alone.

I chat cheerfully to Martin, wanting to keep him distracted and entertained. We all assume that the call to the holding room means that surgery is imminent and that the wait will be of the order of ten minutes. Not so. Ten minutes have passed and then doubled themselves and doubled again. Nearly an hour has gone by. Martin is still fully conscious and I am starting to run out of entertaining patter. Like a comedian about to die on stage before an unforgiving audience, I am desperately searching for material. I sense, though, that the sound of my voice making humorous, inconsequential conversation is soothing for Martin. When I stop, he starts to look restless. And so I continue, improvising wildly on any topic I can catch in passing.

Finally, after what seems like twelve hours but is in reality only one, the nurse comes to wheel Martin into surgery. Amantha and I farewell Martin cheerfully and then, as his trolley disappears into the operating theatre, turn to each other with fear and shock. It is really happening. It is on. And it is completely out of our hands.

We wend our way downstairs to street level. George has said the surgery should take around four hours, and I figure we have a couple hours of wandering through the sunlight and shops before the gravitational pull of needing to be near the centre will tug us back to the hospital.

And so we walk. We stroll, distract each other, and move in and out of the hypnotic colours and textures of the boutiques. And there are ten-minute spaces at a time when we are engrossed in the sensory world of clothing and not thinking about the one that waits outside.

Somewhere around the two-hour mark, the anxiety sets in and refuses to be dislodged. Walking back to the hospital, we can both feel the relentless rise of tension. Our plan is to be in the ICU waiting room from three hours onwards. If things go badly in the operating theatre, time spent in surgery can either be shortened or lengthened. Shortened is the worst possibility – things may have gone so badly wrong that the patient dies on the table. Lengthened is not good either, but at least it means they are doing something and the situation is still viable.

Two hours and forty-five minutes have passed as we enter the hospital car park to pick up some things from the car. Just as we step inside, my phone rings. I feel a jolt of pure terror. I stare at Amantha, whose expression mirrors my own as I scramble to find my phone in the depths of the bag. If it is George, something has gone terribly wrong.

Finally my fingers find the phone and I breathlessly say 'Hello?'

And it is a friend, ringing to see how things are going.

I am in a state of near collapse from the shock of thinking it is George with grim news.

'I can't talk, I can't talk! The phone has to be free for the surgeon'. My voice is coming out in a kind of strangled choke.

It takes fifteen minutes for my heart to slow down.

The ICU waiting room has a couple of couches, a few chairs, some coffee-making equipment and a microwave. A woman is sprawled on the couch, obviously trying to get some sleep, another is flipping through old magazines and a third is rummaging through her bag, about to be an intense nuisance.

Amantha and I settle ourselves down with books and the usual complement of boiled eggs and sandwiches. A family comes in and talks quietly amongst themselves. Very occasionally a surgeon will enter, look to see if the relative they want is there and disappear. Each time the door opens, adrenaline dropkicks me almost to the floor. Is it George? Is it news?

I look around the room, aware that every one of the people sitting here is in the same situation as us. For each of them, something is hanging on a thread, each of them is in an intense, private world of waiting. Each of them, except the woman rummaging in her bag. She has now triumphantly found what she wanted.

Her mobile phone. And she then proceeds to ring what seems like every person she has known in her lifetime and conduct the interminable lost-control-of-the-volume-knob conversations favoured by mobile-phone users in public. The woman trying to sleep stirs restlessly. The rest of us attempt to ignore the intrusive conversation. I keep thinking that surely she will end the call soon and that she must be stressed like the rest of us – be gentle with her.

Finally, after twenty minutes of this and with no end in sight, I get up and politely explain that someone is trying to sleep, that her conversation is disturbing the rest of us and could she please have her conversation outside. I get a nasty look, but she does take herself and her phone out of earshot. The room suddenly feels much larger.

Once three-and-a-half hours hit the clock, the tension, which has already been skyscraper-high, ramps up to the orbit of Pluto. The door opens three times and each time it is as if it has been swung back explosively into my chest. Twice it has opened to admit relatives and once for a nurse. The clock moves to the four-hour mark and suddenly the door swings open again. Someone in surgical scrubs enters. I don't recognise him but then realise he is looking at me. Is it George? It must be George! And I cannot read his expression. I race across to him, too adrenalised to speak.

George nods hello at me. The seconds of silence before his voice makes contact with my brain feel like an eternity. And then, 'It went well', he says. 'We did a repair'.

'Thank you, thank you, thank you!' I have to restrain myself from throwing myself at him in ecstatic gratitude.

And now George smiles. 'He'll be heading to ICU soon. In about an hour you might be able to have a look in at him'. And he heads off back to the operating theatre.

Amantha and I are both weak with relief. Quite literally. My muscles feel as if they have liquefied – my entire body feels as if it has been running a marathon.

'He's fine', Amantha and I repeat stupidly to each other, over and over again in all its tonal variations, 'He's fine!'

We are reduced to burbling, relieved idiots for the next hour. Texting friends to tell them the news is a joy. I want to tell everyone the news. I want to put up a big balloon in the sky with the words in capital letters 'HE'S FINE' trailing after it.

Visiting at the ICU is equivalent to gaining entrance to a high-security secret club. There is a chain of people to be consulted and arcane codes to be used. We start the process at 7.00 pm and finally, at 8.00 pm, the message comes through the door that we can enter.

Martin is the third sleeper on the right. He has tubes coming out of him in every direction and his eyes are closed, but the nurse assures us he has regained consciousness and is doing fine. His heart is beating well and they are keeping him heavily sedated until his blood pressure steadies. Amantha and I lean forward to give him a kiss. I whisper in his ear 'You'll be dancing soon'. I figure that if anything can cross through the drugs, that phrase will. And then we wend our happy way home.

That night, as I am sending my update email, I repeatedly press 'send' only to have my computer refuse to do so. On the fourth unsuccessful attempt, I suddenly realise I am attempting to send the email to 1 October and my computer is staunchly denying that any such person exists.

At regular intervals throughout the night I phone ICU to see how Martin is going. All of these nocturnal enquiries are handled by Martin's night nurse, with whom I am beginning to be on familiar terms. She is a woman with the unique knack of beginning every response with a sentence soaked in ambiguity – able to be interpreted as either he is doing very well or he is doing very badly. This, of course, elicits a sharp rise of stress hormones in the body of the enquirer. As soon as I reply, 'What do you mean?' the nurse then lapses back into more direct communication and says, 'He's doing very well'. I have had four such conversations with her and each time she has managed to start off with a different but equally ambiguous statement. Of course, she may be part of a unique marketing strategy promoted by the Cardiology Department. Each ambiguous response she has given to my 'How is my husband doing?' has certainly had my heart stuttering in alarming ways.

After a night with this mistress of linguistic calisthenics, I am startled on my 7.00 am phone call to get a nurse who quite simply says, 'He's doing really well'. And then offers to put him on the phone. It is beyond exciting to hear his voice, even though it sounds as if he has been woken from a very, very deep sleep.

2 October 2010

We had expected to see Martin awake today, but on all of our visits to him during the day, he is barely up to opening his eyes. We are reliably informed that the physios have had him up out of bed several times (hard to believe) and that he is doing very well. It is equally hard to believe that he could be out of ICU tomorrow as per the original plan.

When I ring at 9.00 pm, though, after getting home, the nurse says George has just been, that he is really pleased with Martin's progress and has confirmed that he can leave ICU tomorrow for a bed on the Cardiac Ward.

I am on my Bluetooth, telling Lynne the news about Martin, when I become aware of a strange, eerie light flashing in the house.

Increasingly concerned, I move cautiously through the house, all the while keeping Lynne posted.

'Is it a police car reflecting through the windows, do you think?' she says.

'No', I reply, 'it's somewhere inside the house. It's weird'.

'I'll stay on the phone while you look', Lynne says. 'Do you have a mobile?'

At which point I realise that what I am seeing is the pulsing blue light of my mobile out of the corner of my eye.

3 October 2010

George's judgement is vindicated. At 2.30 pm, on his second day post-surgery, Martin takes a step upwards in life, from the ICU to the sixth floor Cardiac Ward, and is rolled into his own McMansion of a room – a single room with a view out over the city, and his own bathroom.

He is doing well although still very tired and sleepy. George (who has now attained sainthood in my book) arrives for his visit in the early evening and there follows a delightful exchange between George and Martin.

George: How are you feeling?

Martin: Average.

George: Did you think you'd be running marathons at this stage? Let's start again. How are you feeling?

Martin (smiling for the first time that day): Fine.

And his mood does indeed shift from then on.

4 October 2010

Today Amantha is back at work and I will not have a navigator with me as I drive in. I have carefully written down instructions for the route to the car park, the route within the car park and the route from the car park to the sixth floor. What could possibly go wrong?

The answer to that question comes as I roll into the car park at 9.30 am. A number of other drivers seem to have also picked that arrival time as the magic number. Unfortunately, an even greater number of drivers have picked 9.00 am. The car park is completely full. Many of my fellow 9.30 am entrants are making that discovery simultaneously. A merry chase is being had by all as cars drive into blind alleys, strive to get out of them, jam other cars, honk, curse and honk again.

Finally, dizzy with turning, spinning and backing, I snag a car park that is not strictly there to be snagged and emerge dazed into the hospital for an encounter with the Lawson's dyslexic lifts – you press 'Up', they go down; you press 'Down', they go up. After a lengthy period of riding up and down, I finally make the lift stop at the sixth floor and find my way to Martin's room.

St George has not visited by the time I leave at 4.00 pm, but I might be able to catch him during this evening's visit. All the nurses can tell me about his schedule is that 'He's not an early bird'. When I enquire what this means, they say, 'He doesn't come around at 6.00 am'. How lazy can you get?

5 October 2010

Martin's mood and energy suddenly lift again today, and he is now feeling back to his normal self mood-wise, as well as making rapid progress on the physical front. Yesterday he did three laps of the ward. And today all tubes, wires and catheters are being removed and all is going well. Martin had noticed some blurry vision yesterday but that is much better today – apparently they tell you not to have an eye test for twelve weeks after open-heart surgery, as you may get false results and get the wrong lenses.

I return from buying Martin some grapes to find St George the surgeon paying a visit. He says Martin is doing extremely well and will be out by the end of the week – amazing to think of.

He will not be allowed to go home until he can walk one kilometre. The circuit of the ward is 100 metres, so the goal is to be able to do between ten and fifteen circuits by the time he gets out. Martin, of course, is planning to do fifteen. He says he thinks his day-by-day rate of improvement is exponential rather than gradual. He had already done two laps by the time I got there at 10.00 am.

Update, 5 October 2010

This morning I managed to snaffle the last car park – in a hidden blind alley. The Lawson car park seems to have a number of these (unless I am finding the same one multiple times), and of course by the time I leave the hospital I have forgotten where the car is. I think the circuit around the Lawson car park is significantly more than one kilometre.

In Melbourne the general topic of the day is reliably the state of the weather. In Lawson, the topic du jour *is reliably the state of the lifts. Today Lift 11 was in the naughty chair. It would open its doors seductively, invite people in and then close. And stay closed. And stationary. Its sister, Lift 12, was authoritatively diagnosed with multiple personality disorder – its display lights indicated that it was going both up and down simultaneously. All lifts seem to display symptoms of an eating disorder. No matter what floor you press they will inevitably take you down to the kitchen, where the doors will open and stay open for at least three minutes like hungry dogs at the table staring fixedly at the food they hope will drop into their mouths. New passengers to the lifts become alarmed at this behaviour. Old-timers, a category into which I now place myself, have to reassure them that this is part of normal lift behaviour.*

And the good news is that Martin is now available for visitors. He is on the sixth floor. Don't take Lift 11.

Update, 6 October 2010

The fifth day post-surgery and for the first time there was a blip – Martin had some arrhythmia this morning and his heart rate sped up to 150. He said he knew something was wrong because his heart rate was up and he wasn't dancing. The nurses in the Cardiac Ward monitor all the patients all of the time – the signals from each patient's monitoring equipment are automatically transmitted to the nurses' station, where they are immediately seen and attended to. There was a nurse in Martin's room in a flash.

Martin was given some beta-blockers and instructed to lie down for a few hours. By about 2.00 pm his heart had returned to normal rhythm. It did, however, put a dampener on his planned conquest of the walking circuit, as he was not allowed to do any laps this morning and early afternoon. Nevertheless, he managed four circuits later in the afternoon and evening, and as I walked alongside him I noticed that he was distinctly speedier in his stride than yesterday.

The cardiologist shot in and out to check on him and said that forty per cent of post-cardiac surgery patients get arrhythmia and it is no big deal. This was reassuring to hear, as the nurse has been regaling us with tales of arrhythmia-caused blood clots going to the brain.

St George arrived at 7.30 pm and said that the only surprise is that Martin hadn't got the arrhythmia earlier and that it is nothing to worry about. He is extremely pleased with Martin's progress and says that at this rate he is set to go home on Friday – that is, tomorrow.

Martin is in good spirits and not much discomfort. Although we have heard stories about how painful it is to laugh and cough in the days post-surgery, Martin is finding he can do both without any pain. A cause of greater pain is the daytime TV he has resorted to occasionally watching – he has discovered that it is crap.

On the way downstairs, I took note of the mental health status of lifts 11 and 12. Lift 12 still believes it is going both up and down at the same time. As I passed Lift 11, however, I saw an engineer gazing thoughtfully up at its innards. Lift 11 has obviously been scheduled for some psychosurgery.

Update, 7 October 2010

This morning, as I turned into the Lawson car park after an hour's drive through heavy traffic, the attendant greeted me with the words, 'It's full but you're welcome to try'. Refusing to stop and marvel at the ease with which this man had issued such a perfect double-bind invitation to insanity, I did try. And succeeded. Tucked away in a dark corner of the building, as invisible to the normal eye as Harry Potter's Platform 9¾, was a space just big enough to fit my car.

I emerged into the lobby of the Lawson, decided to try the stairs instead of the lifts and walked straight into a hard, reflecting surface. At this point I realised that I had walked into a mirror instead of the stairs and that my required means of ascent was in fact behind me.

I finally staggered blearily onto the sixth floor at 9.45 am, to be greeted by a sparkling Martin, who had already done seven laps of the circuit.

Martin is in fine spirits, with a hearty appetite and no pain to speak of. I went around the circuit with him (he is now doing double and triple circuits at a time) and said, 'You're walking just as fast as your normal speed'.

'No', replied Martin, 'I'm walking slower because I'm having to wait for you to catch up with me'.

On my way down to pick up lunch, I daringly stepped into Lift 11 and was pleased to discover that yesterday's psychosurgery had worked beautifully. Lift 11 is now a well-behaved member of the Lawson lift community. Its friend Lift 12, however, is not faring so well, and I have had to revise my previous diagnosis. Yesterday I thought it was multiple personality disorder, due to the fact that it was flashing both up and down lights at the same time. Now I believe this was actually a symptom of a manic high and that the true diagnosis is bipolar disorder, as today it is flashing no lights at all.

On my return to Martin's floor, I heard the sounds of raucous laughter shaking the closed door of Martin's room. I entered to the sight of four engineers plus Martin howling with laughter at engineering-type jokes as Martin directed them in the repair of every last three-dimensional object in his room. The leader of this jolly group turned to me and said, 'It's amazing, six previous occupants of this room and no one's ever noticed these flaws before. We love it!'

10 October 2010

Martin arrived home yesterday, just as St George predicted, and is feeling astonishingly good. When we go for our one-kilometre walks around the block, he is only slightly held back by me. St George has ordered two naps a day, though, and Martin is having no trouble complying. He is feeling good – no pain to speak of – and his mood is sunny, in direct contrast to Melbourne's weather. It feels wondrous to have him home, especially knowing that the surreal world of the ICU is only seven days behind us.

15 October 2010

Somebody up there has decided that, removed from the heady excitement of ICU and stuck at home for days in the pouring Melbourne rain, there was a danger we might get bored. He/she/ it has therefore thoughtfully given Martin a spike in temperature. It is a relatively small spike, but to our sensitised ears, it carries a hissing sense of danger.

It is stirring up a case of déjà vu in Robert, Martin's GP, as well. He has instructed Martin to monitor his temperature hourly. That first hour is crawlingly familiar, as the clock slows and we resist the impulse to check Martin's temperature every five minutes. Eventually, the clock arrives at its assigned time and we hold our breath as we remove the thermometer. And breathe again as we see that his temperature has returned to normal. Even so, Robert has scheduled a raft of blood tests for tomorrow morning, so we are still not released from the waiting game.

18 October 2010

Robert rings with the news we don't want to hear. The blood results have come in and Martin's CRP marker is up – he would like to see us in his surgery. The CRP measures inflammation and up is not a good place for it to be. Robert says it may simply be post-surgery inflammation rather than infection that has caused the rise, and that the spike in temperature may have been just a coincidental hiccup. If that is the case, the marker should now start to move downwards. If it doesn't, we may find ourselves suddenly tumbled back into the world of endocarditis.

More blood tests are scheduled for tomorrow and by happy chance we have an appointment with Allan of the IDU on Tuesday, so he will be able to add his expert opinion to the mix.

21 October 2010

Allan's thinking is much the same as Robert's. If the inflammation marker remains raised, we may be in trouble. Another follow-up blood test has been ordered and much will depend on it. The results will be in first thing this morning and Robert has said that we should ring him to get them.

Three phone calls and two hours later, he still has not rung back and I am skittering on the edge of sanity. Finally, after the third phone call, his secretary buzzes him and he sends the message that the news is good, the marker is going down. My nervous system, hauled out of the wrecking yard on receipt of this news, is still protesting a day later.

29 October 2010

Today it is Peter the cardiologist's turn for a follow-up visit. He, too, is extremely pleased with Martin's progress and can hear no murmur when he listens to Martin's heart. All that is there to be heard, Peter says, is the sound of a healthy heart. Without Martin's typed history in hand, there would be no way of telling from his heart sounds that anything had ever been wrong. It is an odd thought – all those months of destruction wiped away, not just to invisibility but to non-existence.

As we walk out of Peter's office, the visit seems oddly, unnervingly, smooth. Too easy, too simple. Every other time we have moved in and out of these doors we have come for verdicts about life or death. The room, the chairs, the floor our feet walk on – all have been weighted with a density of intense, constrained emotion. We have walked in as supplicants, our bodies leaded, our minds tensed to hear the words 'damage, damage, damage'. The strangeness that accompanies today's visit is like the strangeness of a dream where you are skating on a surface that should not sustain you, like an insect crossing the surface of a lake, except that you are not an insect. It is as if safety is at the same time both real and dependent on an illusion.

1 November 2010

More often now I am experiencing long stretches of being immersed in normality – absorbed in enjoying simple daily things with Martin. It feels comfortingly safe and stable until suddenly, with the flick and speed of a switchblade, I am plunged back into the realisation, not just of what *might* have happened, but of what *will* eventually happen. And normality vanishes into the knowledge of death. Sometime. Inevitably. And, as always, it is not my death that frightens me. It is the death of those I love.

Death has usually been a possibility so far off in the future that it is faint with distance – barely an outline visible. Now its existence has been so sharply etched that it feels engraved viscerally. This is what getting older is about. This is what happens. Loss – sudden and irretrievable. Losing the people you love. The people who know you. Being left behind.

I feel like a gadfly. I cannot settle down to things and spend the day starting this, starting that and ending up by finishing nothing. I play with my fabrics and op-shop pieces, see things I can make, startling transformations I can effect, innovations in form and function. I keep seeing new colours, new textures, new fabrics, new ways of combining them. I drop into op shops and fabric shops on my walks, fall in love with the colours, the shapes, the textures. My mind is full of creation after wonderful creation

I have always noticed that when I do not write, I am drawn to creating with fabrics. The sense of joy when disparate colours, textures and shapes come together in unexpected but perfect ways is exactly like the feeling when unpredictable words and images come together in ways that are both entirely new and entirely right. It is the most intense kind of pleasure to see something create itself, even though you are the agent of creation.

A back and neck injury a few years ago meant that I couldn't sit at a computer to write. Simultaneously, I discovered op shops – racks full of colours and textures to play with and prices cheap enough to buy a bundle. The coincidence in time of these two experiences was a deadly one for the house.

Without the ability to sit and write, I was compulsively drawn to fabric. But when you play with words, you need no space at all. When textiles are what you play with, bye-bye dining-room table and every other available surface. I have racks of op-shop clothes growing like wildflowers – fabulous words and phrases of fabric waiting to be cut up and stitched together in gorgeous, unpredictable sentences. It is years before my back allows me to sit at the computer again. And during those years, I have accumulated a lot of fabric.

I also make a startling discovery. As a writer, you never have to let go of your creations. You may sell your works, your words, to a publisher, but they are always there close at hand for you – in your book, on your computer. As an artist – sculptor, painter or textile artist – when you give your creations away, you never touch them again. They belong to someone else. And with this discovery, I realise that as a creator, I am a shockingly possessive mother – I don't want to give my darlings away and never see them again. And so my cupboards are bursting with all the wonderful things I have made and fallen in love with.

I am filled with the impulse to create. The kick of playing with colours and shapes is like a pep drink. Turning this into that and that into something else – marrying two disparate patterns into one startling, new, exquisite whole – gives me a fizz of joy. I have a small insight into what the excitement of mania feels like. And right now, in this driving need to create and keep on creating, perhaps a part of me secretly imagines that if I can keep creating, I can ward off its terrible, terrifying opposite.

Dutifully, though, every day this week I have been going through clothes, sorting, bagging and tossing. But even as I try to tame it, the chaos is seductive – it is only within chaos, after all, that the haphazard and the accidental can meet and catch fire. And so, in mid-toss, I suddenly see a fascinating new way of using this or that particular material – I see if I cut this and shirred that, it would turn into a garment that looked like a fall of leaves. I try it on, I pin and nip. I see what else I need. I rummage through my haberdashery. I find this, the one I have been looking for, but tangled up with it is that, which is even more wonderful. I untangle it, pin it and drape it, find the cotton to sew it. And suddenly I am exhausted and too much time has passed.

There is a constant imbalance between taking up projects and taking out garments I have decided I cannot use. I do regular 'binning' runs through the house – the op-shop-bound bags pile up and are shipped out, but the house never seems tidier. And my constant efforts to make it so are remarkably tiring.

The medical condition of hypothermia, the state of being too cold, passes through a singularly odd phase. As hypothermia increases in intensity and duration, it brings inevitable death. In the early and middle stages, people shiver, huddle, wrap themselves in anything they can find, aware of their extreme need for heat, protecting their bodies. But in the terminal stage, a curious phenomenon appears. It has a name: 'paradoxical undressing'. Those sufferers who are in the final moments of hypothermia where what they most deeply need is warmth, suddenly throw off their clothes as if in the middle of a heatwave.

The medical explanation is that as the body cools to a level it can no longer survive, it gives up trying to save itself – blood is suddenly no longer hoarded to protect the vital organs and instead flows back to the periphery of the body, the extremities and skin, creating a flush of superficial warmth. But to the puzzled observer, if there were one, there would only be the sight of someone insanely, inexplicably and frenziedly doing the exact opposite of what is required for life.

As I rush around creating, creating, creating when what I most need to do is to sit still, I think of this. It is as if the part of me that was in constant motion – fixing, researching, making things happen – the part of me that lived through a time when stillness was danger, has not yet dared to keep up with the other part, the part with its foot in today that is saying, 'It's over. Sit still. You can be still'.

12 November 2010

Today is the occasion of Martin's triumphant return to the driver's seat of his car. This return to driving has become a recurring event to celebrate – rather like a boy having his bar mitzvah, the ceremony that marks the entrance to manhood, over and over again. Each time, however, the thrill is as sweet.

It is impossible to look at Martin today, dancing and driving, and remember that at this time six weeks ago he was being wheeled into the Intensive Care Unit. I am slowly catching up to Martin – my bug is dissipating and incidences of putting socks in the freezer are decreasing – although there is no doubt that were I to be seen in a UK hospital I would be immediately tagged with that wonderful medical acronym NFN (normal for Norfolk).

This morning I have an interesting wake-up experience. A couple of days ago Martin bought a walkie-talkie set. Today, at 6.00 am, I am suddenly woken from sleep by the sound of unfamiliar male voices in the house. As I listen, a man's voice clearly says 'Holy shit!' Martin is still fast asleep – there is no one else who should be in the house.

Like an intrepid fool – one of those idiotic heroines who insists on going down the stairs into the darkened cellar, out into the threatening night, and so on – I get out of bed to investigate. No sign of intruders, but I can still hear voices. Has it finally happened? Have I finally gone around the bend and into the locked ward? And then I see it. Martin's walkie-talkie turned on and rustling with received static. And somewhere out there in the pre-dawn darkness, a man has had something happen to him that caused him to call out 'Holy shit!'

20 December 2010

Martin is recovering well from his cardiac surgery of nearly three months ago. He has come through smoothly, with none of the cognitive or emotional hiccups that can often accompany such surgeries. He is back dancing, walking, doing all of the normal things of daily life. The epilepsy has remained under control. His speech is good, although a little slower and still differently accented to his pre-stroke speech. He can do everything he used to do pre-stroke, just a little more slowly. It is miraculous to look at him now and remember where he has come from. All of his doctors say they have never seen someone come back like this from where he was. It is finally daylight and we have emerged from the nightmare.

I am hanging out for January, when I will take a month off work. Friends have been saying, 'Why don't you go away for a holiday?' And my reply is always the same. For me, a holiday more exotic than any I can imagine is some free time without an impending medical crisis and no responsibilities. This January at home is going to fit the bill beautifully.

A week ago we had been asked to take care of a puppy, a Maltese–Shih tzu cross, for a couple of days before before she travelled on to her new owner. She is due today and I am at home in a fever of excitement, waiting for the arrival of a fluffy, cuddly bundle.

And here she is at last – a fluffy bundle who wants nothing to do with cuddles. In fact, she wants nothing to do with humans. She is in the garden, sitting alertly but quietly and keeping herself a good distance away from us. As I slowly approach, she picks herself up and moves further away. She is not whining, not cowering, not growling, not running – just making sure she keeps metres between us and her. We are told she was kept in a concrete backyard and has never seen grass, and I notice that when she moves, she takes care to walk only on the concrete edges and avoids the grass, which she clearly sees as something foreign and possibly dangerous. Humans also come into the dangerous category for her – it is clear she was abused by one.

I have never met a puppy like this before. The ones I have encountered, even in their cages in pet shops, which I loathe with a passion, have been curious, interested and eager for pats, play and exploration. This little one has the serious demeanour of an orphan who has learned that the world is a dangerous place.

She is four-and-a-half months old. I know puppies go through a fear-imprinting stage from eight to twelve weeks and that some experts say the natural window for human–puppy bonding closes after fourteen weeks. All of her learning in that sensitive stage has been that humans hurt you and must be avoided.

I sit down quietly, a safe distance from her, in the hope that if I do nothing, her natural curiosity may prompt her to move towards me. But she is having none of it. Neither will food or water tempt her. Every time I inch even a little closer to her, she gets up and moves further away. The impasse continues until I simply pick her up and put her on my lap.

She starts shivering with fear. Gently I cradle her and scratch her silky white belly. And then, in a miraculously few seconds, she relaxes into the discovery that this feels good, looks trustingly up at me and asks for more. She has discovered for the first time in her life that humans can be a source of comfort and pleasure. And she doesn't look back. From that moment on, she runs enthusiastically to greet each and every human who crosses her path, certain she loves them and they are going to love her. It is astonishing to see the speed with which all of her previous learning about humans has been eradicated. She is the embodiment of the plastic brain – four months of ground-in learning at a critically sensitive stage, obliterated in seconds. It is as if her brain's natural state is that of an outgoing, trusting being and it has just been liberated. She has been freed to be herself.

I spend hours with her out in the backyard, playing, petting and observing her. So many things are new to her – she has never been within sight of a toy and has no idea what to do with them. Balls, fetching, tug-of-war ropes – all of the usual puppy–human games are foreign to her. She responds to them all with initial puzzlement and cautious interest and then with a resounding 'Yes!'

22 December 2010

I am in love. Despite the fact that I know she will be leaving and I will never see her again, I have fallen for this little white being. Martin is more circumspect – he is not interested in small dogs.

I focus on enjoying the short time with Harriet, as she has been named, and on telling myself she will be going on to a loving home. But when she is packed into her travelling crate for her plane journey, the garden seems empty and I miss her. I really miss her.

Maybe it is now time to get a dog. Martin and I discuss it. One of the issues is that our house is much less puppy-proof than it was years ago when we had our last puppy. Books have spilled over from the bookshelf to a section of the floor. My craft materials are scattered around the house. Impossible to expect a puppy not to be destructive with this cornucopia of temptation around it. I determine for the thousandth time to get a handle on it and set out with renewed vigour on the campaign of ditching, shelving and giving away excess books and fabrics. Realistically, however, I know this is not going to happen fast – work and fatigue have been the murderers of many a good intention. But I persist – maybe we could plan for a puppy a year from now.

24 December 2010

I am out on a walk when my phone rings – the puppy's new home has fallen through. And my heart manages to leap both up and down at the same time. Distress for little Harriet and her long fruitless journey. Hope that maybe we can keep her. Worry that maybe we cannot.

'We'll try and keep her', I say.

This is not the phrase on Martin's lips when I arrive home and tell him the news. 'No', he says. 'I don't want to keep her'.

'But I want to at least give it a try and see if it can work'.

He shakes his head. 'I don't want her and you're too tired. A puppy is a huge amount of work. And it will be impossible to puppy-proof the house. She'll get into everything. You've forgotten what puppies are like'.

But this time, I am just as adamant as he. I plead, persuade, bargain and when all else fails, surprise us both by bursting into tears. 'I really want this', I say. 'You have to give me a chance to see if we can make this work'.

And with this Martin capitulates.

26 December 2010

Harriet is due back this afternoon. For her, it will be a three-hour car ride, a two-hour plane ride and then a further one-hour car drive – a reversal of the trip she took just a few days before – a draining experience for a very young pup.

I rush to the pet shop to buy her a bed, food, toys and all the other things a puppy needs. She arrives home just a few minutes after I do. Her travelling crate is carried to our sunroom and a small furry personage emerges, looks around her and instantly realises she is home.

She bounds up to me and our time with Harriet truly begins.

We are starting from scratch. She has not had her vaccinations, has not been house-trained, has not had any of the usual experiences a nearly five-month-old puppy should have had. The vet pronounces her fit and healthy and she licks his hand after he has just given her an injection. The gesture is pure Harriet. She loves the world.

I am already madly in love and within a few days, Martin has joined me in that delirious state. And it just grows. I have loved all of my dogs. I thought at the time that I loved them as much as it was possible to love a dog. When they died, I wept on and off for weeks as I encountered the missing greeting, the place where they should have been sleeping, the jarring absence when my hand reached out to stroke them, the loss of a loved member of the family.

I thought I knew what it was like to love a dog. Harriet is showing me I didn't. I find myself sitting next to her on the floor, stroking her silky head and saying in the tones of foolish, doting lovers, 'I love you, I love you'. There is something so captivating and complex about her personality that it reduces Martin and me to strings of repetitive superlatives that invariably end with 'Isn't she amazing?' We are the most besotted of besotted puppy parents.

And Harriet really is very special. Our last two dogs were standard poodles, routinely considered to be in the top three most intelligent breeds. But Harriet runs rings around them for intelligence. She doesn't have an aggressive bone in her body but she is spunky and stands up for herself. She adores us and loves to be with us but is totally relaxed when we leave her behind in the house. She thinks things out for herself and when we begin training, she learns easily but believes in the work-for-a-wage principle. Treats will do the trick. Praise she enjoys but doesn't need. It is as if she is so sure of our love and her secure permanence in the pack that praise packs no extra punch for her. She is obedient and loves us dearly, but it is because she chooses to, not because she needs to.

And most amazingly, without needing to be told, she knows exactly which articles on the floor or within paw or jaw reach are hers and which are ours. And she simply doesn't touch ours. The one exception is a book titled *Dog Tags* with a photo of a golden retriever on the cover. I discover it sitting neatly next to the pile of books on which it was placed with one bite, complete with tooth-shaped jagged edges, neatly taken out of the bottom right-hand corner of the cover. At first I think it is an ingenious part of the cover design. Closer examination, however, reveals the bite was executed post-production. It remains the only object not belonging to Harriet that she has marked.

It is hard for me to write about Harriet without degenerating into the voice of a Hallmark card. As if everything to be said about a dog's love and the love for a dog has the sound of cliché or soppiness. And yet it is all true. A hundred times a day, Martin or I will stop, smile and pet her or throw balls for her. If you could measure joy in millilitres, jugs and jugs of joy are drunk by us each day because of Harriet. She is so obviously her own little person – totally devoted, totally loving but with her own interests, her own quirks, her own big, celebratory personality.

I had forgotten just how much of a sentient being a dog is. Harriet is extraordinarily pretty, a chocolate-box cover of a dog, but what we are in love with is that elusive phenomenon about which I have been musing through Martin's stroke and Faith's shape-shifting – her own unique and deeply rooted way of being in the world, her personality. I watch her extrovert delight in greeting strangers, her adventurous embracing of new experiences – qualities that seem such core aspects of her personality – and I remember the shy, cautious puppy that steadfastly refused to let anyone near her. And I wonder sometimes what would have happened to Harriet if she had gone to a different home without loving humans or a secure pack. Who would she have been?

And for the first time with a dog, as I sit with her stroking her fur or scratching her freckled tummy as she and I gaze into each other's eyes, I think of mortality. Harriet is full of energy, a lover of fun and chasing games, her coat a thick silk of white with honey patches. She exudes health and exuberance and yet sometimes as I sit with her, I am struck through by the thought that her life is likely to be shorter than mine. That it is probable that I will face the experience of losing her.

That is true, of course, of all the dogs I have lived with and loved, but never before have I thought it. And I am taken suddenly back to decades ago, when I first read the Gerard Manley Hopkins poem about grief and loss 'Spring and Fall: To a Young Child'. The poem opens with a young child grieving over the falling leaves of autumn and ends with the recognition that loss and death are an inextricable part of being human. When I first read it as a young person who had not known loss, I loved it for its words, images and rhythms but was somehow not emotionally touched by its subject matter. Now it rings sonorously and beautifully through my head as I stroke Harriet and realise that all we have is now, now, now.

14 January 2011

Every silver lining is said to have a cloud and the massive silver lining that is Harriet carries with it a tiny cloud that stems from her first weeks with us. Anyone who has owned a puppy knows that those first weeks are reminiscent of the first weeks with a baby – full of sleepless nights and constant watchfulness. Harriet's first few weeks are no exception.

Not for the usual howling that is common in a pup's first few nights away from its mother, but because Harriet has taken her guarding duties seriously since her first day with us and in her self-appointed role as security officer, she has decided that the possums in the backyard are invading our territory. As the local possums also take their garden rights very seriously, there is a natural clash of interests. This results in several loud barking episodes per night. In the interests of Martin's sleep, as well as the neighbours', I am up several times a night to let Harriet know possums are not a threat. After two long weeks, Harriet finally accepts the possums, or at least most of them, as enfranchised occupants of the garden and settles down.

Not so my body. My thyroid has had an up-and-down relationship with the thyroid work ethic over the last thirty years. It has regular go-slow periods where it dips below normal. Not dangerously so, but enough for me to feel the symptoms of a sluggish thyroid with great clarity. It has been behaving itself for a few years now, but with the January rest I was hanging out for turning into two weeks of no sleep and the constant on-call needs of a new puppy, my thyroid once again downs its tools.

The symptoms are familiar in their unpleasantness and include the tendency to fall asleep whenever I sit down, even after Harriet and I are back to sleeping through the night. I stagger rather blearily on, hoping my thyroid will right itself in time. But it clearly has no intention of doing so. My GP confirms what was already clearly evident to my body – that my thyroid is out of balance. She prescribes a little thyroxine and I head back home with high hopes.

The thyroxine gets my thyroid back to within normal limits but unfortunately the symptoms are only slightly eased. I decide a holiday might help my body get back in balance and I pencil out ten days without patients where I can simply relax at home with Martin and Harriet.

30 June 2011

I have now had two attempts at clearing ten days off for a holiday. On the morning of the first attempt, while Martin and I stood chatting with a fellow dog-owner in the dog park, I found my face suddenly zooming down to meet the ground. Not even a second's notice to allow my hands to buffer my fall.

When I painfully clambered back into a vertical position, I discovered that a large black dog had bolted straight through the centre of our triad, bashing into my knees, and that I had flown over its head to land flat on my face on the ground. My nose was bleeding, my face was battered and I had broken a rib. Only the sponginess of the wet grass had saved me from more serious injury. I spent my holiday painfully recuperating.

On my next attempt, two months later, to clear time for a holiday, the scar tissue from my ovarian cancer surgeries decided to imitate Velcro and twist my bowels around. I avoided hospitalisation by the skin of my teeth and spent the rest of my holiday painfully recuperating.

Ever optimistic, I have cleared out another ten days, two months later. I have avoided dogs in the park. I am very careful about stressing my innards. The weather is even likely to be good. What could possibly go wrong?

Four letters. BRCA.

Part 4

When I was first diagnosed with ovarian cancer in 1994, the discovery of a set of gene mutations in what came to be called the BRCA genes was still a work in progress. The mutations disable the protective mechanisms of these genes so that women with these mutations have a far higher risk of getting cancers of the breast and ovaries than women without the mutations.

By 1996, when I had a recurrence of ovarian cancer, researchers were exploring the association of the genetic mutation, which came to be called BRCA1, with the incidence of cancers in the women who carried it. It was the beginning of decades of discovery and the unveiling of knowledge that was as terrifying as it was beneficial, as debilitating as it was empowering.

My first encounter with the BRCA gene came through a friend. During the time of my ovarian cancer recurrence, I had joined an online support group for women with ovarian cancer. It was in the relatively early days of the internet, and the group was small, intimate and based in America – I was the sole Australian.

There were some truly wonderful women on the list and we formed a close bond, emailing each other off- as well as online. I am one of the few survivors of that time, and the memory of those women is as rich and real to me as if it were yesterday. I have never been able to bring myself to delete their email addresses from my computer. In some other universe, they are still alive and, were I to type in their address and press send, I would receive their familiar responses.

Anna was one of the women in the group. She was a paediatrician working in a city at the epicentre of cutting-edge cancer research in America. She was an exceptional person – intelligent and warm, funny and caring. When my hair fell out, Anna sent me a wooden comb to remind me it would grow back. I still have that comb in my drawer.

Quite soon after Anna's treatment for ovarian cancer had finished, a pilot study was being organised to test women for the presence of the BRCA1 mutation. Anna decided to take part in it. Anna drew the genetic short straw – she had the BRCA1 mutation. She wrote to me, talking over the decisions to be made. Then as now, the only two alternatives offered were prophylactic mastectomy (where healthy breasts are removed as a preventative measure), or an oestrogen-blocking drug (tamoxifen in this case) and surveillance.

At that point Anna thought she would eventually opt for the prophylactic mastectomy but figured she had time to make the decision. Her ovaries had already been removed in the surgery necessitated by her cancer and she thought the chemo regime she had just come off, added to the absence of ovaries, would give her a few safe years in which to make a decision. She was in her early fifties.

A few years went by. Anna had been taking the tamoxifen and getting regular breast scans. She had recovered well from the ovarian cancer and was planning to go to Africa to do some work as a paediatrician with the children there. She wanted to give back. She was all set to go when she wrote to tell me she had been diagnosed with breast cancer. Soon after she completed her chemotherapy for breast cancer, she had a recurrence of the ovarian cancer, eight years after the initial diagnosis. She was fifty-eight when she died.

Further news of the BRCA gene filtered through slowly over the years. There were more and bigger studies. Two more mutations were found. These three mutations – two on the BRCA1 gene and one on BRCA2 – became known as the founder mutations. Descendants of the Jews of Eastern Europe, the Ashkenazim, are at particular risk of carrying these faulty genes. If one of your parents has the mutated gene, you have a fifty per cent chance of inheriting it. If you have the gene, each of your children has a fifty per cent chance of inheriting the gene. Males can carry the faulty gene as well as females.

Estimates vary but the BRCA1 mutations are believed to carry with them an up to eighty-seven per cent lifetime risk of breast cancer and a forty per cent lifetime risk of ovarian cancer. The BRCA2 gene similarly carries a high risk of breast cancer but a lower risk of ovarian cancer. Making the decision to be tested for the BRCA gene mutations is to open yourself up to powerful knowledge, the impact of which can be both devastating and healing. It is information, too, that once known can never be un-known. It is knowledge that impacts not only upon you but upon your children and your whole extended family.

When the test became available in Australia, I put some thought into whether I should be tested. I'd had ovarian cancer at an early age, a strike against me (genetic cancers tend to arrive earlier than their sporadic cousins) and I was an Ashkenazi Jew, a second strike. On the positive side, there was no family history of either breast or ovarian cancers. However, to modify that, there was very little family history at all – both my parents' families had died in the Holocaust. They had not lived long enough to get those cancers. My mother had died of cancer of the pancreas at the age of sixty-three, a cancer thought at the time to have no association with the BRCA genes, my sister has never had cancer and my father also has never had cancer.

I clearly had a chance of having the mutated gene, but equally clearly also had the possibility of being free of it. And, importantly, Amantha was only twenty. She had not had children, and the only reliable way of preventing ovarian cancer is to remove a woman's ovaries – a huge and devastating thing for a young woman who is yet to have children.

Some of the cancers that affect women have screening processes that can be used to monitor women at risk and pick up the cancers while they are still in the early stage. Breast cancer risk can be responded to with increased screening – ultrasounds, MRIs and biopsies The Pap smear can detect potential cervical cancers even before they have properly evolved. Ovarian cancer, however, is another thing altogether. To date researchers have not come up with a screening method that is reliable, has high predictability and will consistently pick up early ovarian cancer without confusing it with benign cysts or causing collateral damage via the diagnostic process.

Without the security of an accurate screening test, carrying the knowledge that you are at risk of developing ovarian cancer is a hugely stressful experience. Ovarian cancer is the most deadly of the gynaecological cancers. If caught early, it has an excellent cure rate. If caught late, as most of them are, the survival statistics are far from good.

Ovarian cancer used to be called the silent cancer because its early symptoms were invisible. Now it is often called the cancer that whispers. The symptoms of early ovarian cancer are often present but they are subtle and mimic the benign maladies of everyday life – bloating, gas, indigestion, heartburn, expanding waistline. Sometimes there are more unusual symptoms, such as feeling full more quickly than usual after eating, pelvic, abdominal or back pain and extreme fatigue, but these symptoms are often pushed aside as muscle pain or the effect of an overly stressful lifestyle. Too often women, and sometimes their doctors as well, treat what they are observing as the hoof beats of the common horse when really the sounds are that of the uncommon zebra of ovarian cancer.

Without a way to prevent or pick up this deadly cancer in its early stages, women at risk are living in the shoes of Damocles – that character from myth who looked up from the throne where he had to spend his days only to see that poised directly above his head, and suspended from the ceiling by a single thread of horsehair, was a giant sword.

I wrestle with the impossible decision of whether knowledge for Amantha at this stage is good or bad. And, of course, I cannot even ask her whether she would prefer to know or not, because as soon as that question is asked, the knowledge of the terrible possibilities is opened up and cannot be shut down again.

In the end I decide not to take the test. Amantha has not yet reached the age where oncologists feel she is in real danger – I decide that for her to have the knowledge at this stage would involve needless stress. There will be time enough to stress when she is a little older. In addition, I am guessing that my chances of not having the gene are higher than those of having it.

All one can do in a situation like this is walk the highwire of mathematical probabilities, each choice point potentially deadly. Every woman must make her individual decision with the understanding of how she would cope and what she would choose to know or not to know. And of course for parents, the choice is often made on behalf of children – an even more wrenching decision. I make sure I counsel Amantha on the importance of breast examinations and that she knows to watch out for the early signs of ovarian cancer, and then all I can do is let it go for the moment.

A few years go by. I have been keeping my eye on the research coming out about the BRCA genes. It is coming through only in dribs and drabs, and the picture has seemed unchanging until one day I read with a shock that cancer of the pancreas is now thought to be associated with the BRCA gene mutations.

I sit up. I now have three ticks instead of two – I have been tipped into a higher risk category. My mother is a first-degree relative and the fact that she died of cancer of the pancreas is now definitely relevant. Amantha is older now and in a settled relationship; she could handle the knowledge. It is time for me to open the box.

I decide to have the test without telling Amantha. That way, if the test comes back free of the mutation, she will have been saved months of worry. If it turns out I have the mutation, I will tell her then and we can work through what she needs to do together. I ask my oncologist how to go about getting the gene test and he gives me the name of a hospital hosting the Familial Cancers Unit.

I ring and discover that it takes weeks, even months, to get an appointment. Somehow, having gone through the long, intense process of decision-making, I have imagined that once the decision was made, the rest of the process would be fast. Nothing is fast, I am about to discover, in the world of BRCA testing.

I have been reading about the BRCA gene – in scientific papers but also first-person accounts. The first books written by women who have the mutation are starting to come out. Months ago, I ordered one of these online, expecting it would be delivered within a week, but it has been absent from my postbox. The book, *Pretty Is What Changes* by Jessica Queller, has been garnering many articles and glowing reviews. Its author is a young woman who discovers she has the BRCA gene mutation and is forced to come to terms with this deadly heritage. I have been looking forward to reading it, but it is more than two months since I ordered it and it clearly doesn't seem destined to reach my mailbox.

The day of the long-awaited appointment with the genetic counsellor finally arrives. Just as I am about to get into the car, I notice that the post is in and, with my lifelong inability to resist pouncing on the mail with hopefulness as soon as it arrives, I get out of the car to retrieve it. A handful of letters and a parcel. The letters are just the usual array of bills. The parcel contains a book: *Pretty Is What Changes*.

The Familial Cancer Unit is set in the middle of an oncology unit. Walking through it stirs up memories of my stints as a patient in an oncology unit. People are everywhere – on their way to appointments, coming from appointments, waiting for appointments. Looked at from a distance, these people in their normal street clothes with mostly neutral expressions on their faces might be everyday shoppers at a mall. But no one is here for everyday reasons. By the very fact of needing to come here, you have stepped across the line society defines as 'normal'. As I walk past the various clinics, I think to myself that if grief and pain were colours, the air would be opaque with them.

My genetic counsellor introduces herself and leads us to a small interview room. She explains what is currently known about the

BRCA gene and says that after taking my history they will be able to give me a rough idea of the likelihood I may be carrying the mutation. If there is a reasonably high risk of my having the mutation they will then expect me to go away and think about whether I want to have the test.

The three ticks on the 'risk' boxes I knew about – early age of onset of ovarian cancer, mother with cancer of the pancreas and Ashkenazi origins are indeed weighted as risks. As for the rest of the family history that can tell so much about genetic predilections, it is missing. The counsellor says she will go off and consult some figures to give me an assessment of my situation – that is, the probability that the genetic mutation runs in my family.

After a short while she arrives back with some papers in her hand and says 'We've assessed you as having a risk factor of forty per cent'.

The experience of hearing a hard figure – actual numbers after so many weeks of vagueness and wonderings is startling. The forty per cent, I realise, is higher than I thought it would be, but it doesn't seem overwhelmingly high.

Some years after my recurrence of ovarian cancer, I came across a study on women who had experienced a similar recurrence to mine. At the time of my recurrence there had been no studies that were relevant – my presentation was somewhat unusual and it had taken researchers time to find a large enough body of women to study. As I read the research, I was chilled to discover that in fact, at the time of my recurrence, I had only a twenty-four per cent chance of being alive five years from then – that is, a seventy-six per cent chance of being dead. So, in comparison, while forty per cent is a sizeable risk, at the same time there is the greater sixty per cent chance that I am free of the mutation.

In addition, I am used to thinking of BRCA families as having clusters of breast and ovarian cancers. In my family I am the only one who has had ovarian or breast cancer. Surely that means I am unlikely to have the defective gene. What I don't know yet is that clusters of these cancers are not always present in families with the mutations. In some families the mutation expresses itself (through a cancer developing) only occasionally.

The counsellor has said to think it over and if I decide to have the test, to give her a call so that she can arrange another appointment and then the blood test. It is 2009, near the middle of the year. I am just about to phone for an appointment when we go dancing in Frankston on a Saturday in early June.

Martin's stroke and the cascade of continuous medical crises over the next two years sideline everything else. It is mid-2011 before I am able to stop and draw breath.

4 August 2011

Martin is doing extraordinarily well, far exceeding anything his doctors predicted. His speech is good, his epilepsy is under control, he is back dancing, doing his woodworking and other hobbies. He is able to do everything he did pre-stroke, including complex computer programming. He had returned to his work as a computer analyst part-time after his stroke but retired a few months later, before his cardiac surgery, and is relishing spending time with his hobbies. He is a little slower than he used to be in doing some things, but as he was exceptionally fast previously, this deficit is not a problem.

One day my friend Davida phones from America. Davida, like me, has had ovarian cancer and its associated chemo cocktail. For her as for me, the chemo, although lifesaving, has left a legacy of reduced energy. This is a common after-effect of our particular chemo, and when I ask my oncologist how long it lasts, he says that for many women it never goes away – the latest research is confirming that the lasting fatigue is in fact due to subtle physiological deficits left by the chemo. Both Davida and I seem to be in that category.

When Davida rings, Martin answers the phone and they chat, Davida asking how Martin is.

'Fine', he says, although he notes with frustration that he is slower at doing things and gets tired more easily.

'Join the club', says Davida.

Afterwards, Martin says to me that for the first time in the fifteen years since my last cancer diagnosis, he understands what I have been describing. But that apart, he is flourishing. He is fit, healthy and has enough in the way of hobbies to keep him busy for the next millennium. Harriet is a constant delight and we are both head over heels about her. I am back seeing my normal caseload of patients and looking forward to January, when I will take a month off and luxuriate in the freedom of no work, no medical crises and plenty of sunshine. The storm is over.

The only to-do thing left on my medical plate is the BRCA blood test. I ring to make an appointment, imagining I will be able to walk straight in and take it.

'But I've already had a counselling appointment', I explain to the receptionist who tells me I need to make another counselling appointment.

She is unswayed. It seems I have to go through a repeat counselling appointment before I can then have an appointment for my blood test.

This time around I have told Amantha I will be having the test and asked what she would like to do. Amantha is very clear about her course of action. She wants to be tested. She wants the knowledge. Not everyone does. It is highly loaded knowledge and many decide they are not ready for it – that it would prove too stressful or they would be unable to undertake the approved preventative measures and the knowledge would be a constant source of anxiety.

Amantha decides to have her test at the same time as I do. I ring up to book our dual appointments and immediately run into the problem with that particular plan. Due to the expense of the test, the gateway to it is carefully guarded. If I prove to be free of the mutation, then Amantha is at no risk and her test will have been unnecessary. We will have to proceed single file, Amantha waiting until my test results come through before being allowed to proceed with her own.

And so I go ahead with my counselling appointment and blood test. It is the simplest of experiences – you walk into a room, a nurse draws a small amount of blood, labels it and you go home knowing that nothing may be the same again.

The wait for the results of the blood test is long. Two months long, they tell me at the hospital. My third attempt this year to clear two weeks off for a break falls just before the end of that period. Good timing, I think. I will be able to catch some R and R before the results come in.

15 September 2011

A week before my third-time-lucky holiday, I get a call from the Familial Cancer Centre – my test results have come in early. I have an appointment to go in and have a counsellor give me the results.

The tension returns with a whoosh. Why have the results arrived three weeks earlier than expected? Is that a good sign or a bad sign? I have absolutely no idea. I daydream about how wonderful it would be to go in there and be given the all clear. And a holiday to follow with no medical weights on my mind. As I imagine it, I can feel the relief, I can feel the lightness. I can feel the freedom.

My unconscious mind is feeling neither relief nor freedom. I dream I am on the Melbourne University campus – I am standing outside talking to Amantha, telling her I cannot remember where I have parked my car. I am holding two bags, one in each hand. I put my two bags down for a second to pick something up and when I straighten up again they are gone. Someone has stolen them. I am devastated. I have no keys, no money, everything is gone and I have no way even of getting home. I ask Amantha for her phone to ring Martin for a lift but his phone is on message mode and I cannot get through to him. Despite my distress, however, Amantha seems fine – unflustered and self-possessed.

I wake up with the ominous feeling that my unconscious mind is trying to tell me something. That I do have the mutation. That the two bags that are whisked away represent my breasts and the prophylactic mastectomy. Everyone's dreams have their own symbolic language – when the setting of any of my dreams is a university campus, I know my unconscious mind is trying to tell me something serious.

Nevertheless, I keep hoping. All the way out the front door, where I note to my amusement that Fate, in the form of the post office, has decided to repeat its synchronicity trick by arranging for a second long-delayed book on the BRCA gene to be delivered to my doorstep on the day of my genetic counselling appointment.

I keep hoping all the way into the city and all the way through the snaking corridors that lead to the Familial Cancer Centre. I am hoping as I sit down in the waiting room and am called in to see the counsellor. I am hoping all the way up until the counsellor opens her mouth and tells me I have the mutation.

As soon as she has said it, it becomes real. 'And that explains', she says 'why you developed ovarian cancer at such an early age'. And I am thrown back to that search for explanations in Martin's illness. The 'why, why, why' his doctors were continually chasing. It seems quietly amazing that all these 'whys' do have answers.

The counsellor goes on to talk about the various options available to me. Various is overstating it, of course. There are still only two options. Exactly the same two options that were available to my friend Anna a decade and a half ago – surveillance and oestrogen-blockers or prophylactic mastectomy.

My mutation is in the BRCA1 gene. Breast cancers in BRC1 women tend to be classified as triple-negative – they are particularly aggressive and particularly hard to treat as many of the drugs in the current breast-cancer armoury don't work on them. Among other things, triple-negative tumours have no receptors for oestrogen. As tamoxifen works by blocking oestrogen from cancers that use it to grow, I wonder why an oestrogen-blocker is useful for a tumour that has no oestrogen receptors.

When I ask the counsellor this, she shrugs. 'It's a good question', she says. 'The answer is that at this point in time we just don't know'.

In a couple of years from now, further research will in fact emerge suggesting that BRCA women who have already been diagnosed with breast cancer stand a significantly lower chance of a second cancer if they take tamoxifen. This beneficial effect held whether the tumours were oestrogen-receptive or not. For now, however, all the counsellor can tell me is that although they are not totally sure of the mechanisms involved, they recommend oestrogen-blockers for BRCA women who do not have mastectomies.

The counsellor then reaches into a folder and brings out a page of columns and graphs. 'These are the risk assessments for BRCA1 mutations', she says.

The columns represent the lifetime risk a woman has of getting breast cancer if she has the BRCA1 mutation. Studies have come up with varying lifetime risks of BRCA women developing breast cancer – some of these suggest that the risk is as high as eighty-seven per cent. This translates to the woman having only a thirteen per cent chance of *not* getting breast cancer.

The counsellor continues, 'That risk factor is over a lifetime. I calculate that because you've reached sixty, you've outlived a significant portion of the risk. Most of these women get breast cancer in their forties'.

I am unconvinced. These studies are lumping a whole pile of women together – there must be other factors that differentiate the women, and their risk, more precisely.

'What about the women who get ovarian cancer first? At what age do they tend to get breast cancer?'

'We don't know', she says. 'No one's done the studies'.

I am not surprised by this answer, not only because this whole area of research is relatively young but because most women who get ovarian cancer don't live long enough to get breast cancer later on. By now, though, I know two BRCA women who have had ovarian cancer first. Both of them discovered their ovarian tumours at a slightly older age than I did and both developed their breast cancers some years later – at, or just under, the age of sixty.

Two patients do not a study make, but as they are the only two women I have ever known with both ovarian cancer and the BRCA mutation, they definitely make a mark in my mind.

The news that you carry the BRCA mutation immediately brings with it the question of what you are going to do with that knowledge. You will have had that gene for all of your life, but if you have not known about it, this one moment of revelation changes everything.

Many women choose surveillance over a prophylactic mastectomy. They don't want to lose their breasts unless they have to. The thinking here is that surveillance will pick up the cancer early when it is curable. And of course there is a chance they may never get breast cancer at all. Why sacrifice healthy breasts and undergo major surgeries until forced to do so?

The cons of this approach include the possibility that the breast cancer may not be detected early enough and some cancers, even though detected early may still come back to kill. And the triple-negative breast cancers, as well as being particularly aggressive, are also difficult to treat and are more likely to have spread before detection. In addition, if a cancer is found, you may have to go through chemotherapy and radiation and perhaps have a mastectomy in less than ideal circumstances. You will also have to live with the uncertainty engendered by a diagnosis of cancer – will you have a recurrence? As well as this, even if you never develop breast cancer, the regular screening means frequent periods of stress and tension while waiting for results and, for many women, the sense of living with the constant presence of danger.

Prophylactic mastectomy, which means having your healthy breasts removed, is a huge step. As well as the trauma of losing valued and visible parts of your body, it involves major surgeries, most often two major surgeries – the first usually covers the mastectomy and initial stage of reconstruction and the second surgery completes the reconstruction. It is hard enough to go through this kind of surgery in the wake of a breast-cancer diagnosis when the need to remove cancer-ridden breasts is clearly evident. To make the decision to have a mastectomy while your breasts are healthy and there is a chance they may stay that way, is daunting indeed. For some women a prophylactic mastectomy feels unbearable and unimaginable while for others it feels difficult but doable. On the pro side, it reduces the risk of developing breast cancer to extremely low levels, below that of women who don't have the BRCA mutations. The sword hanging over your head is to all practical purposes cut down and stowed away.

From the beginning I have been sure that if I have the mutation, I will take the prophylactic mastectomy route. I have had two encounters with ovarian cancer, I am not enthusiastic about making the acquaintance of another member of the cancer family. I am extraordinarily lucky to be alive today – statistically speaking, my recurrence should have finished me off years ago. I am not interested in pressing my luck. The counsellor's statement about having outlived a lot of my lifetime risk has made me stop and think, though.

I am used to statistics – they are an essential part of a psychologist's training. I understand the notion of lifetime risk in theory but I just cannot seem to apply it to myself in these circumstances. Martin feels the same. He, too, is very familiar with statistics, but neither of us can get our head around this particular issue. I head off to Dr Google to do some searching.

I am following up my thought that the faulty gene expresses itself differently in different women. Why, for example, does it result in ovarian cancer in one woman and breast cancer in another? The answers to these questions are still up in the air – no one knows. I am searching, though, for studies that look at whether outcomes are different for women who are first diagnosed with ovarian cancer. Just as the counsellor said, I cannot find any of those. Then I have another idea – there are three founder BRCA mutations; perhaps someone has looked at whether there is a difference in what happens to women with each of these mutations.

After a fairly lengthy search, I finally find it, a study that separated women into groups of each of the three mutations and looked at the average age of onset of breast cancer (technically known as the penetrance of the gene) for each. And lo and behold, my particular mutation, 185delAG was different from the other two – the median age at which my mutation resulted in the emergence of breast cancer was fifty-five, with a confidence interval (of ninety-five per cent) reaching up to the age of fifty-nine and a half. The median is the number that sits in the middle of the range of ages at which the women were diagnosed with breast cancer. The fact that the median age was fifty-five implies that about fifty per cent of 185delAG women may contract breast cancer after the age of fifty-five.

Because the number of participants in the study was limited, the researchers could not be sure of the precise median, but they can be ninety-five per cent certain this median lies somewhere between the ages of 46.7 and 59.5. So, although unlikely, it is possible that fifty per cent of women with the 185delAG mutation will contract breast cancer even after the age of fifty-nine and a half.

For the other two mutations, the median ages of breast cancer diagnosis were forty-seven and forty-one – significantly younger than my mutation's median age of fifty-five – and the researchers concluded that women with the 185delAG mutation seem to be diagnosed with breast cancer at a significantly older age than those with the other mutations.

And so, according to this research, with fifty per cent of 185delAG women likely to develop breast cancer after the age of fifty-five, I may not have outlived the majority of my risk – it is possible that I am right in the firing line.

It is only one study and I cannot find any that have tried to replicate its findings, but it is enough to settle any lingering doubts aroused by the counsellor's comments. I am clear on what my course of action will be.

That, of course, doesn't mean I am happy about it, but I am clear about what I need to do for me. And that is a huge blessing. For many women, as well as the terrifying news that they have the genetic mutation, there is the extra hell of going backwards and forwards in their mind about what to do.

What I am feeling right now for myself is probably best described with a gesture – that age-old, eyes-rolled-upward, 'Well, for heaven's sake, what next?' snapshot of body mime. I am shocked and weary but not devastated, weeping or terrified. This news comes on the heels of two years of nonstop life-threatening crises for Martin – the BRCA news pales in comparison. I am not sick and I don't have cancer. I know what cancer is like – at least this way I get a chance to avoid it. All my concern right now is focused on what this news means for Amantha.

Everything is experienced in, and takes its meaning from, a context – and for me that context is probably relatively unusual. When I get to talk to, and read about, women in the throes of post-test BRCA discovery, many of them are grieving and shattered. Some have already been diagnosed with breast cancer and have this news coming on top of that. Others are young, and the impact of losing their ovaries and breasts is horrifyingly magnified compared to those who already have children or who have passed menopause. Others have no supportive spouse to help them through. Every one has her own unique circumstances and her own response to the trauma, and I am in a relatively lucky position.

I start telling friends, both about the test results and that I plan to have a prophylactic mastectomy. With only a few exceptions, their responses run along the lines of 'Isn't that too extreme? Why are you rushing into this? Why not wait until you have to? Isn't there something else you can do?' They are worried for me and aware of the enormity and irrevocable nature of the surgery I am planning. Repeatedly, I have to go through the odds and the extraordinarily high lifetime risk of getting breast cancer and ask them if they would get on a plane that stood a near ninety per cent chance of crashing. That is when they understand.

The smaller group, who agree with my decision immediately, include the genetic oncologist, who, when I ask her, says that is what she would choose, too. Further down the track, my GP spontaneously ventures that this is what she would do as well. And when I tell Cindy, she immediately says, 'I'm selfishly pleased that you're doing that. I want you alive'. Martin and Amantha trust my judgement and are wholeheartedly behind me – they want me to do whatever gives me the best chance of being cancer-free.

Having made the decision, I want to implement it, get it over with so I can be clear of it. I am experiencing what many women who have the gene and have had to go through repeated call-backs and biopsies experience – the sense of living with the ticking time bomb.

I went through this, of course, after each of my cancer diagnoses. Cancer survivors have to learn to live with the uncertainty of recurrence. It is one of the many challenges of a cancer diagnosis, and all you can do is try for the best balance between keeping an eye out for relevant symptoms and not being obsessed by them. It is not easy but it is all there is. Up until now, of course, I have not been aware that my breasts have come under the time-bomb category. Now that I know, I want to defuse that bomb as soon as possible.

As always, there is research to be done. Do I want reconstruction or just a mastectomy? For me it is a definite yes for reconstruction. What kind of reconstruction? There are different types, there may be options.

And there is also the team of surgeons to pick. For a mastectomy and reconstruction, you need both a breast surgeon and a plastic surgeon. My GP is away on holidays, so I don't have a medico to ask about that. I go back into the old phone-a-friend routine I had to perfect when I was micro-managing Martin's medical treatment. I read articles and books describing the different techniques. And I also find the FORCE website.

FORCE stands for Facing Our Risk of Cancer Empowered and it is an Aladdin's cave of treasure for anyone needing support or knowledge to do with the BRCA gene mutations. It was founded by an extraordinary woman, Sue Friedman, who was determined that no one should have to face what she faced alone.

It is a wonderful resource and I type in its web address several times each day as I think of more and more questions.

19 September 2011

I have been trying to get a message through to my sister. I want to let her know I have been tested and to ask if she wants to know the results for her own medical interests. I have her son's email address and have sent him an explanatory message. It takes a couple of emails and then he replies to tell me that Lily had the test years ago and won the genetic lottery – she does not carry the BRCA mutation.

And, of course, the next utterly terrifying step is to get Amantha tested. I will have inherited the BRCA gene from my mother. As with any child of a parent carrying the faulty gene, I had a fifty per cent chance of inheriting it and fifty per cent chance of being free of it. Lily and me, my mother's two children, landed neatly on each side of the fifty per cent divide. Like me, Amantha has a fifty per cent chance of landing on the wrong side of that line. I cannot bear to think of it.

Amantha phones for an appointment, but as usual nothing happens fast. She has to wait for an appointment with a counsellor and then she has to wait the six to eight weeks for the results of her test. It is sheer, undiluted agony. I am suddenly struck with the useless bit of hindsight that if I'd had the foresight, as opposed to its backwards sibling, I could have organised for Amantha to be tested first. With a grandmother who died of cancer of the pancreas, a mother with early onset ovarian cancer and an Ashkenazi Jewish lineage, she would have been able to pass through the gateway before me and we would have had her results by now. I can understand the need to limit expenses with this testing, but the practical impact of having to wait like this is excruciating.

Although I am calm on the surface, I am in a continual state of inner dread in the lead-up to Amantha's results. My dreams are not. They have been arriving with a colourful array of settings and characters but the theme is the same – there is danger around, but

Amantha is safe. Things get lost or stolen but are returned intact. They are stressful, but not nightmares. There are threatening circumstances but things work out. It is startling that my tension is not reflected in night-time dreams of terror. I am not usually given to 'wish fulfilment' dreams – a Pollyanna-ish denial of real and oncoming danger. I just have to hope my unconscious mind knows something that I don't.

I occupy myself during this time with the search for the right surgical team for me. It is, if not a pleasant distraction, at least a time-consuming one. I have the names of three excellent breast surgeons. My plan is to see them and choose one. I also have to line up plastic surgeons, see them and choose one. Then I have to make sure the breast surgeon I choose works with the plastic surgeon I choose. If they don't it is game over and back to the beginning.

I finally narrow it down to two teams – Carol and Jim or Julie and Bill. I have appointments with them all, some further off than others. This morning, however, after hearing good things about Carol and Jim, I decide I will go with them. My task today is to see if they a) work at the same hospital, and b) work together. There follows a morning on the phone playing Hospital Cluedo – Dr Carol in the library with the knife? Dr Jim in the study with the dagger? Can I get both Dr Carol and Dr Jim together in the kitchen with their chosen sharp implements?

These telephonic experiences include a lengthy, mutually puzzling conversation with the receptionist of a totally different surgeon when I accidentally ring the wrong number. I finally work out that Carol practises in the Lawson and York hospitals but that Jim practises at Burke. I am just about to give up in despair when I say to Carol's receptionist that it is just that I was trying to match my plastic surgeon with my breast surgeon and she says, 'Who is your plastic surgeon?' I say 'Jim', and she said 'Oh, Jim. No problem, Carol will go where Jim is. They work together regularly'. Relief! So it is now Carol and Jim in the kitchen with the dagger.

Having decided this, I phone to cancel my appointment, a couple of weeks hence, with Julie, the breast surgeon from Team 2.

Exactly fifteen minutes after I have done this, I get a phone call from my friend Lynne, who tells me she has a friend who has the gene and has had a recent prophylactic mastectomy and that she would be happy to talk to me. I ring Lynne's friend. She is very generous and helpful with her comments, says her results are fantastic and that her breast surgeon is terrific and a wonderful person. I enquire after the name of her surgeon and it is Julie, whose appointment I have just cancelled.

Back to the drawing board. And to the phone. Julie's reception-ist sounds slightly puzzled. 'But didn't you just cancel your appointment?' Needless to say, the appointment I cancelled has been taken up, so I have to wait longer to get the next available one.

Next task is to snaffle an appointment with Bill, the plastic surgeon of Team 2. Not so easy. He is booked out and then going on long holidays. My anxiety level begins to rise. I really want to get a date. It is nearing the end of the year – too late to have it done this year – and I really want to have it over with as early as possible in the New Year so that it is not hanging over my head, which is starting to spin with the pros and cons of Carol, Jim, Julie and Bill.

7 October 2011

All through this time, my GP has been away on holidays so I have had no one with whom to talk things over or who can suggest referrals. She was due back a couple of days ago and I have an appointment with her this morning. I have had to juggle the times around to fit in with my work commitments, but I have been looking forward to seeing her and talking through my decisions. I turn up at her rooms, complete with a carefully written-out list of the names of the specialist referrals I need from her.

I walk up to the receptionist's desk and she looks at me puzzled. 'Your appointment was for yesterday', she says.

I look at her blankly.

'Yesterday', she repeats. 'At eleven'.

Somehow, in all the juggling of times, names and everything else going on in my head, I had managed to imprint the wrong time for this appointment. I was so sure of it I hadn't even bothered to check my diary before leaving the house. 'Are there any free spots today?' I ask.

The receptionist shakes her head. 'I'm afraid we're totally booked out. The next free space is next week'.

I apologise for the missed appointment, thank the receptionist, walk outside and burst into tears. It is only then that I realise just how much I have been yearning to talk my decision-making over with someone who knows the ropes, to not have to micro-manage and make every decision alone as I'd had to in those first months of Martin's illness.

I am feeling better by the end of the day. I have appointments lined up with my new chosen team of Julie and Bill, and I should be able to schedule the surgery for early March next year. Amantha has her initial session with the genetic counsellor this week, so the eight-week wait for test results will begin.

10 October 2011

On my visits to the FORCE website, I am beginning to recognise the names and personalities of various regular posters on the message board. The posters are split between newbies who are just starting the process, or are midway through and need advice and support, and those more seasoned, who have been there and done that and are offering what the newbies need. It is such a comfort to have somewhere to post the most trivial or serious of concerns and get responses from people who have travelled the same road.

One of the things I quickly get to realise is that surgery for a double mastectomy and reconstruction of the type I will be having leaves you pretty incapacitated for a few weeks. There are two main options for reconstruction – one is flap surgery, in which fat from another part of the body is used to reconstruct the breasts, and the other involves silicone or saline implants. Although I would love to be able to avail myself of flap surgery, I am pretty sure I don't have enough fat for that and will have to go the silicone-implant route for reconstruction.

With this particular kind of surgery, you are not allowed to lift your arms above shoulder height for two weeks, and using your pectoral muscles for the first week or two is a wistful dream. As we use our pectoral muscles for an extraordinary number of everyday actions without even noticing, their absence comes as a rude shock. Try getting out of bed from a prone position without using your arms as leverage. Try opening a jar or turning a tap. Suddenly you will appreciate those dependable unsung pectorals. The word coming down from the women who have been there is 'Prepare yourself to be absolutely helpless for the first couple of weeks'.

While browsing the web for information, I come across a news item from a US paper about a woman whose friends have thrown her a party on the evening before her prophylactic mastectomy. She wears a T-shirt, across the chest of which is printed 'Shhh. Don't tell them. They don't know yet'. I laugh and think, 'What a great attitude'. A couple of hours later, I suddenly think, 'I bet she doesn't have daughters'. I go back to the website and read more closely. And yes, although she has children, she has no daughters.

Daughters and mothers are what make this one of the cruellest of genes. One researcher writes that it is the gene that produces motherless daughters through the generations, striking at women after they are old enough to have become a mother, killing them before their daughters are grown and then repeating the cycle.

14 October 2011

My appointment with Julie, the breast surgeon of my chosen Team 2 is coming up. I have cancelled the appointments with Team 1 and am settled with my Team 2 decision. Now it is just a matter of meeting the two surgeons and finalising the date for surgery. Julie's meeting is first.

It is a warm day and I have on a brightly coloured summer dress. And then, on an impulse, just before leaving the house, I reach again into the cupboard for one of the colourful headbands I have made, to which I have pinned a mass of bright fabric flowers. It comes complete with dangling fabric plaits on which are pinned more fabric flowers. It makes me smile every time I wear it, and people regularly stop me in the street to say they love it. It is riotously gorgeous, full of colour and fun. It is, however, also conspicuous. Very conspicuous. And not the kind of outfit that usually turns up in breast surgeons' offices.

I am experiencing what seems a near compulsion to wear it. It feels important. I don't analyse it; I just put it on. I am a dazzle of colour with my bright cotton dress and vivid cotton flowers framing the headband and bouncing around my shoulders as I move.

Walk through the streets in this outfit and people smile at you. Walking through the hospital, however, I am struck by a lack of reaction – no one is looking at anyone else. The one exception is a woman coming out of the lift as I am stepping in. She takes in my outfit, grins and gives me a thumbs-up sign. 'I could be friends with that woman', I think. We have responded to some essential part of each other.

Julie, bless her heart, manages to not blink an eye as I walk into her office. She knows I am a psychologist who has worked for a long time with oncology patients. Now she also thinks I am a lunatic.

It is not until some time afterwards that I think about this urgent need to wear that particular outfit to that appointment. In part it was because I wanted to walk into that surgery, to meet that experience, head high and singing. As I cannot sing, the colours do it for me. And also, it was the same feeling I had years ago while sitting in the office of an oncologist I had never met, knowing I was about to be diagnosed with a deadly cancer. I had a sudden, urgent need to go through that experience as 'me'. I knew back then that I was going to lose a number of things precious to my identity, including possibly my life – it felt imperative that whatever else I lost, I should not lose myself. And these colours, textures, flowers, shapes that I love creating with fabric are a core part of me.

Julie lives up to her reputation. She is communicative, competent and thoughtful in her answers to my questions. In my childhood, some of the books I swallowed whole were the Enid Blyton series.

The Magic Faraway Tree left an indelible mark in my heart, but Blyton also wrote several series of boarding school stories – *The Malory Towers* series, the *Naughtiest Girl in the School* series and the *St Clare's* series. In *St Clare's* there is Doris the Dunce. And in *Malory Towers* the Doris is described as 'too pious for words'. Sadly, this coloured my appreciation of my name for a number of years. The only other character from all those school stories whose name I remember is Hilary, the steady, super-competent girl we meet in the first book who becomes head girl of St Clare's by the second-last book. As I leave Julie's office, I realise that I have just met Hilary.

17 November 2011

After weeks of trying, I have finally scored an appointment with Bill, the plastic surgeon. Flushed with the success of the hunt, I get a rush of excitement when the receptionist actually says he can fit me in. I feel almost elated and have to remind myself I am getting excited about getting an appointment to meet someone who is going to cut off my body parts.

Bill is businesslike, courteous and efficient. I go through my list of questions and he confirms my suspicion that I don't have enough fat to be a candidate for flap surgery and adds that even if I did, the scars from my two ovarian cancer surgeries would make it impossible, so it is the silicone route for me.

But, most amazing of all, I leave the office with a date, an actual date for the surgery. It will be early March, a time I have picked carefully so that it falls between school holidays – the surgeons will not be away and I may even be able to have my second surgery over with before my birthday at the end of June. Oddly enough, the timing of these surgeries will cover almost the identical dates, displaced by a few years, to those covered by my chemotherapy for ovarian cancer.

And as I continue my reading on the BRCA genes, I find another item related to time that takes my breath away with a kind of wonder. Researchers focusing on my particular mutation, 185delAG, have discovered it can be traced back 2,500 years – to the time of the second destruction of the Temple – when the Jewish people were driven out of Jerusalem and exiled to Babylon. Some part of me goes all the way back in time in a straight line to that faraway place and those ancient people of history and legend.

22 November 2011

With still a couple of weeks to go before her results were due, Amantha unexpectedly received a call from the Familial Cancer Centre to say that her results would be in early and that she had an appointment with the counsellor in a few days to receive them. Tension immediately ratcheted up to inner-screaming level. And still my dreams remained positive. In dream after dream, the child or young animal in the dream remained safe even though there was danger around.

Time has been slowing in the approach to the counsellor's session. Hours have ground by as effortfully as if I were actually having to push them. There has been no escape, even through my usual sanctuary of books. Finally, the morning has arrived. Amantha heads off with her partner for her appointment. I head off to my computer, desperate to distract myself.

During my time on the FORCE discussion list, I have become friendly with one of the regular posters. Eva is a talented singer–songwriter and cabaret artist in Seattle. A few days ago, she started a limerick thread on the FORCE message board, explaining that limericks were one of her ways of managing stress. It is received with delight – with women writing, reading and laughing instead of crying.

I, too, am a fan of limerotherapy. As I sit there waiting for the phone to ring, I scribble one off and post it on the site.

> I'm waiting right now for my daughter
> to ring with results that will sort her
> from BRCA or none –
> still the phone hasn't rung
> and I think I may burst an aorta.

I have just seen it appear on screen when the phone rings. My heart nearly stops. And then I scream aloud with joy. It is Amantha and she doesn't have the gene.

I walk around all that day smiling and laughing like a lunatic. Nothing else seems important. My daughter doesn't have the gene. She doesn't have to live in fear. She doesn't have to make those terrible, wrenching decisions. She is free, free, free!

6 February 2012

Adhering to my usual Boy Scout principles, I set about preparing for the hospital stay. FORCE has a wonderfully useful list of what to take to hospital on its website. It includes button-through nighties. An easy-to-find item, I think blithely. Wrong. Somewhere, some clothing manufacturer's fortune is waiting to be made when they discover the heretofore hidden niche market of button-through nighties for hospital stays.

After much fruitless searching, I end up with a number of homemade variations, including some made from men's shirts. Ditto for the silk pyjamas also recommended – they help you slither along via bum-shuffling in your attempts to sit up or shift position in bed without using your pectoral muscles.

I read all that I can about the upcoming surgeries. I read informative manuals, memoirs, message boards, anything I can get my hands on that is relevant. I want to know what will happen. I want to know what it feels like. I want to know how people cope. I post questions on the FORCE board and respond to others. I access it three and four times a day. It is a lifeline in those weeks when I am the only person I know about to embark on this journey.

I also find my attention regularly drawn to women's breasts – in the street, in magazines, on the screen. Not something that has happened to me before. But, just as when you are pregnant, or wishing to be, you see pregnant women everywhere, I am seeing breasts. Wherever I go, there they are. My gaze is not prurient in any way, rather it is like that of a sculptor's – I see shape, size proportions. I appreciate the beauty. And with it comes a wistful sense of loss.

But I am also planning a Bye Bye Boobs Party for the week before my mastectomy. I invite thirteen special female friends. The invitation runs thus…

> You are invited to join Doris for a Bye Bye Boobs Party in a morning of fun, laughter, games, trivia, prizes and delightful company!
>
> Please bring:
> 1) Yourself.
> 2) A plate of finger food (and if the food is boob-related, so much the better (e.g. scones with a cherry on top).
> 3) The best joke you know, or have heard/read/looked up on the internet.
> 4) And if you're game to share – the time you made the biggest booby of yourself or the story of your biggest boo-boo.
>
> Dress code: As this is an occasion dedicated to choosing life, come in 'the outfit you wouldn't be seen dead in'.

A plaintive query is received from one friend re the eminently rational concern that as she does not purchase outfits she wouldn't be seen dead in, her choice of outfits for the party is limited. In response, a legal loophole of interpretation is offered: 'In addition to an outfit that you wouldn't be seen dead in, you may also (if pressed) wear an outfit you wouldn't be buried in because it is so spectacular that surviving family members would rush to snatch it up before said burial'.

To ensure that these are indeed outfits no one would be seen dead in, I purchase a bundle of extremely cheap and exceptionally colourful bras from a brand-new bin in the op shop to do double duty, so to speak, as headgear – they make stunning tiaras. Although these create an eye-popping drop-dead effect, they are certain not to be adopted as standard burial wear.

The entertainment includes breast-orientated quizzes. (What size are the largest recorded set of breasts? Answer: In early 2009, Sheyla Hershey of Brazil was awarded the Guinness World Record for having the largest set of breasts. After nine surgeries and more than a gallon of silicone, her breasts are a size 38KKK.)

Among the prizes for quiz-winners are, of course, two booby prizes for the losers. And as well as the jokes, boo-boos and quizzes, I have also organised a variant of the 'Pin the Tail on the Donkey' game – 'Pin the Nipple on the Booby', artwork skilfully executed by Amantha.

I have a lot of fun planning the party, with its associated quizzes, prizes and games. It will be the ideal laugh-inducing antidote to an unpleasant experience.

10 February 2012

My visits to the FORCE website with its BRCA-related discussion literature has introduced me to the acronyms that are a universal part of any online discussion list. Back in the days of my ovarian cancer online group, posts often referred to dancing with Ned (NED – no evidence of disease). Newcomers would occasionally post puzzled queries about who Ned was and why everyone wanted to dance with him.

On the FORCE list, the most used acronyms are PBM (prophylactic bilateral mastectomy), BSO (bilateral salpingo-oophorectomy – the removal of ovaries and fallopian tubes) and Da Vinci (not the artist, but the robotic technique used for the BSO). As I browse, I start to notice another regularly occurring acronym – NOLA.

I am puzzled by this. Is NOLA related to NED? I notice that, as with NED, a lot of people want to get together with NOLA. I am just about to post and enquire when someone does it for me. NOLA, it turns out is FORCE-speak for the New Orleans–based Centre For Restorative Surgery. This is the universe's centre of excellence for breast reconstruction. Once I start noticing the word NOLA, it pops up constantly.

In post after post I read of women who consulted several breast and plastic surgeons and were told that they did not have enough fat to create new breasts or that scars from previous abdominal surgeries would make it impossible. They then go to NOLA and emerge triumphant with the breasts they were told could not be created. At NOLA, the loaves and the fishes seem to be alive and thriving.

In America, it is legally mandated that all aspects of reconstructive breast surgery for breast cancer or BRCA women be covered by insurance. For many women, this top-of-the-line surgery at NOLA costs nothing and for others whose insurance is mostly tied to other hospitals, there is often a way of negotiating things so that out-of-pocket fees come to a few thousand dollars. If a woman were to go to NOLA without any American insurance, it would cost upwards of US$100,000. It is ironic that we in Australia, with our excellent health system, cannot offer what this American system offers for women who need reconstructive surgery. There is no NOLA equivalent in Australia and I, who have private insurance, will nevertheless end up paying a very hefty amount of money out of pocket for what is medically, as opposed to cosmetically, driven surgery. I am lucky – I have the ability to work longer hours to pay for it. So many women don't.

Given a win in Tattslotto, I might be heading off NOLA-wards. As the win has not eventuated, NOLA has been relegated to fantasy. As with any good fantasy, it has a siren-like lure. Up until I discovered the superpowers of the NOLA surgeons, I had understood from my surgical consultations here that it was simply not possible for me to have flap surgery with breasts constructed from my own natural tissue. I had accepted that it would have to be silicone for me. Discovering that NOLA could do it differently has stirred the pot, however, and I spend several spread-out hours of useless time thinking 'If only…If only…' I read the posts of the countless women glowing about their stunning post-NOLA results and think, 'If only…' I sneak longing peeks at the NOLA website and think, 'If only…'

Finally, I dream I am at NOLA. I cannot get the surgeons I know do the brilliant work there. Instead, I am given a surgeon who is young and inexperienced. I feel immediate discomfort with him. In the distance, I can see the real surgeons standing with their arms resting lightly on the shoulders of their successful patients-to-be, gazing out into the sky and spouting off worthy spiritual quotes. Even in my dream, I think, 'This is ridiculous'.

I wake, realising that my unconscious is rapping me over the knuckles and saying, 'Get a life!' Enough fantasising about NOLA.

21 February 2012

It is now only three weeks to my surgery and I have been busying myself organising my hospital couture. I have decided that what I want around me is people who are laughing and smiling. To that end, I have opened up my stacked drawers of rubber stamps and am creating fabric badges from some of the most amusing to sew onto my hospital nighties.

Samples include:

- 'Calories (noun): Tiny creatures that live in your closet and sew your clothes a little bit tighter every night'.
- 'If at first you don't succeed, so much for skydiving'.
- 'If a man is talking in the woods and there is no woman to hear him, is he still wrong?'
- 'I'm weird but I'm saving up to be eccentric'.

And also, appropriately positioned, the perfect rubber stamp for this occasion: 'You are now entering The Altered Zone'.

3 March 2012

It is my Bye Bye Boobs Party today. The breast-shaped menu has been entered into enthusiastically, with friends bringing a variety of appropriate foods. Amantha has been helping to create breast-oriented quizzes – the store of esoteric information out there relating to breasts is astonishing. The bra-tiaras have been perfected and the prizes wrapped. All that remains is to have fun. And we do.

It is a riotous morning. The 'Bring your biggest boo-boo' segment is a particular hit, the highlight of which is the following tale.

On holiday in a foreign country, my friend is cruising the stalls in a local bazaar. Spying an item she wants to look at and at the same time seizing the opportunity to practise her fledgling grasp of a foreign language – she knows how to name this object – she gestures to the man lounging behind the counter and speaks.

His eyes open wide and he regards her in amazement.

Pleased with the impact her impeccable pronunciation has had on him, she repeats her request.

The man gapes. Slowly he begins to move forward.

And suddenly her friend grabs her arm and tells her what she has actually said: 'I want to see your penis'.

They turn tail and run. The excited chatter of surrounding stallholders follows them. 'She wants to see your penis! Hey, she wants to see your penis!'

13 March 2012

Suddenly it is surgery day. Pre-admission, Amantha and I go for a walk in the autumn sunshine. I am feeling calm. I have made my hypnosis tape for the surgery. I have done all that I can do. I will come out on the other side of this – it is time to let it happen.

I have not had the lead-up reactions of tears or extreme anxiety that are so commonly described on the FORCE discussion list. And, as it turns out, I will not have the equally common reaction of extreme relief afterwards. I will wake simply feeling glad the surgery is over. I have been lucky not to have been living with the dread of breast cancer for years, as so many of these women have, so I don't have the intense relief of having all those years of anxiety lifted from my shoulders.

I am fortunate, too, in that I don't have to worry about the complications of lymphoedema or irradiated skin. And I have also had the experience of facing this kind of surgery knowing that I did in fact have a very nasty form of cancer. This is so much easier.

Unwished for, of course, and highly unpleasant but, from my particular perspective, far from the worst thing that has happened to me in these last three years. This is perhaps the one advantage of having experienced those years – another of the fabric stamps I have sewn onto my nightie reads: 'Swallow a live toad first thing Monday morning and nothing worse will happen to you for the rest of the week'. I am hoping I have already swallowed my live toad.

This hospital has the policy of ushering patients straight up to the operating suite. With my previous major surgeries, I was admitted as a patient and then taken to my room where I changed into hospital clothes and sat in bed, awaiting either an overnight stay before surgery or the arrival of an anaesthetist to take details and give information before my transport on a hospital trolley upwards or downwards to the sanctum of the operating suites.

It is somewhat disconcerting to be ushered straight up in my 'civvies' to the suites surrounding the operating theatres, a little like being told you can vote before going through your citizenship initiation ceremony. I cannot help feeling that I have not been inducted properly. Being made a citizen of the hospital surely requires you to have changed into the national costume, been given your own bed and laid claim to it before going through the country's more intense rites of surgery.

But apparently, informality is the inductive code of the hour. The relevant questionnaires were filled in downstairs. Up here, I change into a hospital gown and hop on the trolley that will take me to theatre. A pair of pulsing leggings are rolled up onto my legs, where they clench and relax like an unnaturally worried pair of moonboots. Covering my body is the amazing inflated doona through which heated air streams to keep me cosily warm. Every bed should come equipped with one of these.

The cubicle's thin curtains are regularly parted by a stream of surgery-related visitors making their introductions. The anaesthetist, the surgeon, the surgeon's assistant, the surgical nurse. I had no idea I had invited so many people. I begin to feel like the guest of honour at a very large party. And then, finally, it is my turn to be rolled in. The usual magic needle wielded by a smiling anaesthetist. And then I am waking up. In my own room. A full citizen of the hospital.

My memories of post-surgical pain are limited to my two ovarian cancer surgeries, both of which required a procedure called a laparotomy and extensive excavation and removal of my innards. The surgery was major, as was the pain. This is what I have been expecting when I wake from this surgery. But it is not there. I am sore, certainly. In pain, certainly. But not extreme, nothing like the post-operative pain of my ovarian cancer surgery. This really excites me. I develop a bad case of hubris and start snortily turning up my nose at the pettiness of this pain. When Julie comes in to visit, I tell her to her astonishment that compared to my previous surgery, this is a picnic.

What is not a picnic is manoeuvring myself around. Everything I have been told about helplessness is true. Shifting my position in bed by even a centimetre requires a massive and extended effort. Bum-shuffling is the order of the day and I begin to develop retrospective respect for newly ambulatory babies.

I have tubes coming out of several orifices and am attached to drips as well as drainage bags. Any venture out of bed involves several minutes of bum-shuffling to situate myself towards the upper end of the bed, strange rocking motions to get my recumbent self into the seated position, and then extensive searches for the two drainage bags so that I can carry them instead of moving on without doing so and inadvertently ripping them out of my body.

My first night is spent in the hospital patient's version of 'Are we there yet?' Every half-hour I turn on the light, look at the clock and subside, with great difficulty and equal measure of despair, back into the endless time of the sleepless.

Amantha has bought me a Kindle as a present but either she has forgotten to instruct me in its use or I have forgotten that she has instructed me in its use. I suspect the latter. Similarly, I have borrowed Martin's iPad as a source of in-hospital entertainment but I know I have forgotten his instructions. They seemed so simple at the time that writing them down hardly seemed worth it. And just as I think this, I remember that the sensible part of me understood that for me, writing down the instructions for any form of techno-feat was not only worth it but essential. I scrabble around and finally find the instructions, only further to find that I don't understand them. I bum-shuffle back into the infinite hospital night, made even more bitter by the knowledge that just inches away from me lies a feast of books if only I could unlock it.

Finally, the clock tells me it is heading towards 5.00 am. Morning is declared and I turn the lights on permanently and spend a fruitless hour alternately inspecting the iPad and the instructions I have scrawled down. Nothing seems to correlate. I press various buttons and let my fingers tap-dance across its surface, but the iPad is doing what I could not – remaining soundly asleep.

Eventually, the distraction of breakfast clatters its way onto my tray-table. The chef has obviously been practising for the *MasterChef* reinvention test, taking that old stalwart of breakfast toast and reinventing it as Wettex. Even the addition of a heavy layer of Vegemite fails to disguise the true nature of its host. The milk, in turn, has the strange, watered consistency of milk reduced to powder, reliquefied, redried, diluted with seven parts of dishwater and poured into the hospital elegance of a miniature steel milk jug. The jug is probably tastier than its contents.

And then Amantha arrives, smiling and full of energy and able to induct me into the mysteries of the iPad and the Kindle. She has also brought a moving montage of Harriet photos as well as a photo of Martin, Amantha, me and Harriet for my bedside table.

The room, in the light of a new day, is still as large and spacious as I remember it. I am also delighted to discover that, tucked away in a corner of the room, is a large, multi-jointed reclining chair. Once I find the position in which I can sit comfortably (a devilishly challenging task), this chair will become the object of my intense and unadulterated passion.

At first I assume that every room has a chair like this. In my perambulations around the ward, however, I discover that no, I am the only one. I make discreet enquiries about the origins of my chair and am told that it belongs to the Day Oncology Unit.

'I don't know how it found its way here', the nurse says with a puzzled air. And I realise immediately that this chair is on the run and that it is my bounden duty to hide and shelter it. Sheltering is easy. Hiding, not so much. It is a very large chair. But I do my best by keeping my door shut and my recumbent form draped over the chair.

On the fourth day, however, these ruses fail. I arrive back from one of my exercise walks around the ward to discover my chair being wheeled away by a large authoritative nurse. I am distraught and spend the next forty-eight hours doing everything except printing its photo on cereal packets in an attempt to discover its whereabouts. Nothing works, until suddenly my missing partner mysteriously materialises again in its familiar old corner. We do a one-sided version of the old slow-mo crescendo of lovers sighting each other across a field. And the slo-mo need not be technically feigned. This is how I move naturally post-surgery.

But each day I am moving faster and for longer. The pain meds I am on are working brilliantly and all I can feel is discomfort. Not the euphemistic discomfort of doctors about to attempt some unpleasant medical procedure but discomfort as distinguished from pain. The drips are out and my attention is now focused on the drains. They are my last impediment to freedom and getting out of hospital. They have to reach a stable low before it is deemed appropriate to remove them and they are refusing to do so. I have been hoping to leave hospital after a week, but on the sixth day both Julie and Bill tell me that I will need another few days in hospital.

The next morning as I wake wondering whether 'a few' means two, three or four more days, I overhear a conversation going on outside my room. A voice says snappishly, 'We need another bed'. The second voice murmurs something I cannot catch. The original voice, with even more snap in it, suddenly looms closer to my door and snarls, 'What's she still doing in here?'

I am about to discover that the owner of the snappish voice is the head nurse for the day and she is determined to get rid of me. While not averse to her plan, I am aware that both of my surgeons told me just yesterday that I needed a few more days in hospital.

She stares at me aggressively. 'You don't need to be here. Nurse', she gestures to a passing slave, 'take those drips out'.

'Don't you think you should ask my surgeons?' I venture.

She snorts at me and picks up the phone to ring Bill. 'Your patient is ready to leave', she announces to Bill. 'We just need you to look at her'. The thunk with which she puts down the telephone translates as, 'And don't even think of disagreeing with me'.

Within minutes Bill has arrived, my drains have been removed and I am in the car heading home. Within more minutes, I am back in the car heading to hospital, having developed a bad case of leaking drain incisions. Re-bandaged and stocked up with a supply of sanitary pads to do the work the drainage bags were doing, I am back home again, delighted to be in my familiar surroundings, even more delighted to be reunited with Harriet and about to discover that the gods have not forgotten my dismissive hubris of the first week. I am about to experience pain.

It makes itself felt as the morning pain medications I ingested at the hospital for breakfast wear off. I take the Panadol the nurse has suggested and wait for some relief. No dice. The pain is chortling at the very idea.

By evening I am exhausted. I remain continually amazed at just how tiring the simple move from hospital to home always is, and this move is running true to form. I am tired but I am also in serious pain and it is clear that like an attention-seeking and loquacious guest, the pain is not keen on my consciousness removing itself to sleep.

I take a sleeping tablet and eventually drift off, only to wake two hours later with the pain shaking me by the shoulder, irritated that I have nodded off while it was speaking to me. It is clear that there is to be no more sleep for me tonight. The 2.00 am house is dark and silent. I bum-shuffle my way out of bed and into the recliner chair with a book to which I attempt to pay attention throughout the long, long night.

But hey, it's only my first night home. It's bound to get better, right? Wrong. Day after day, the pain continues relentlessly. The best way of describing it is to imagine that you have been very severely sunburned and are now forced to wear a barbed-wire bra on top of the sunburn. The pain has a particularly strident quality that I have never experienced before. It is nerve pain and I am immediately struck by the horror of those patients for whom nerve pain is a permanent condition.

On my dressing-change visit to Bill's nurse, I mention that the pain has been very intense and is not abating. She looks unconcerned. 'Try Panadeine Forte', she says. 'That's a bit stronger than Panadol'.

The pain is as amused by Panadeine Forte as it was by Panadol. I soldier on. After a few more days, the soldiering turns to staggering on. It is now nearly three weeks post-surgery and the pain is as intense and continual as ever. I had started with the happy assumption that whatever it was at the beginning, it was bound to get better day by day.

This pain, it seems, however, has no intention of easing up. I begin to feel an odd sense of claustrophobia about it. It is all-encompassing, all-enveloping – what if there is never an exit door? As each day appears out of yet another sleepless night, the passage of time begins to blur. A quality of being dislocated in time and place takes over – I am anchored and boxed in by the unending, unwavering pain. There are no modulations in it – it is like a voice shouting in my ear in exactly the same monotone without once stopping to draw breath. It is so different from what I expected. I cannot understand why the pain is not diminishing. And I begin to wonder if it ever will.

And then, two weeks after my homecoming, I have my follow-up visit with Julie, the breast surgeon.

'Oh', she says in response to me telling her the pain has been steadily intense. 'Isn't the OxyContin working?'

'What OxyContin?' I say.

'You were supposed to leave hospital with OxyContin twice a day'.

The things they forget to tell you. OxyContin is a major painkiller. It is what I was on during my hospital week and accounted for my breezy passage through it.

Julie is angry. 'This is not acceptable', she says. 'I'm going to give them a piece of my mind'.

And looking at her furious face, I melt. It feels so good to have someone on your side and fighting for you.

I return home from Julie's with a prescription for OxyContin and luxuriate in my first night's sleep for two weeks. And then Eva writes to me in a response to my last email griping about the never-ending pain. Her surgeons at NOLA have given their patients pages of information of the 'What to expect' kind. This is in stark contrast to the skimpy postage-stamp-sized leaflet given to me, which states that mastectomy does not usually involve much pain – a statement that had me turning the colour of an eggplant.

The NOLA surgeons tell you that not only is there pain but that in a counterintuitive fashion it actually starts getting worse instead of better during weeks three to six until very suddenly, at around week eight, it starts to feel better. Other women on the list also write in to say that they were in more pain at week three than they were at week one. It is enormously reassuring to discover that what I am feeling is normal.

With my silicone implants, I have opted for a two-stage procedure. This means that during the mastectomy, some expanders were placed under my pectoral muscles and semi-filled with saline. The amount of saline will be gradually increased in order to stretch the skin and muscles preparatory to the insertion of the permanent silicone implants. I have woken from my surgery with 200 millilitres of saline already in my expanders. They have the softness of boulders, are somewhat square and have the rather unnerving, and definitely irritating, quality of extruding into my underarms. Having just finished rereading *The Hitchhiker's Guide to the Galaxy*, I am in the position where I can keep reminding myself that at least I am not Eccentrica Gallumbits – the Triple-Breasted Whore of Eroticon Six. I suspect, however, that, Eccentrica or not, if I live to be a hundred I will never get used to the sensation of breasts under my armpits. All I can do is sincerely hope that when the temporary expanders are removed, with them will go my underarm protrusions.

It is also time for my first 'fill' with Bill. This involves being blown up like a party balloon. Bill finds the port under my skin in the expanders, puts a syringe in and fills them with more saline. My pain management takes a sudden step backwards for the next few days in the aftermath. And, irritatingly, I am also larger than I want to be. I need to have some of the saline taken out. This is eerily like those segmented books of childhood where if you turn one section of the page, this head appears on that body. Turn another page and a different body appears on that head. I am not used to having my bodily outlines change at the press of a button.

On the positive side, however, I have now been allowed to return to the dance floor. I can lift my hands up over my head, I can drive, I can wash my hair to my heart's content and am seeing patients again. In two months I will return to surgery to have the expanders swapped over to the permanent implants and also have some nipples created.

12 June 2012

The two months have come around fairly quickly. Everyone says that this swap-over from expanders to permanent implants is an easy recovery compared to the original surgery. And despite the fact that it is two-and-a-half hours of surgery (the previous one was four-and-a-half), it is indeed much easier. I am only in hospital for three days and the pain is only a weak imitation of its elder sibling. I am still restricted to sleeping on my back, but that has been the case since my first surgery three months ago – it is still too painful to sleep on my side.

8 August 2012

I have been wrapped in tapes and bandages, to which my allergic skin has been protesting violently, but at last it is time to stop being an Egyptian mummy. The nurse unpeels the various layers of bandages and adhesives and I head home to the mirror. And dismay.

One side is perfectly fine but the other side looks as if it has been in a fender bender – ridges and dents are prominent. 'Perhaps they will round themselves out in the manner of dented foam', I think wistfully. Foam, alas, is not their role model. The dents and ridges remain. I see Julie the breast surgeon for one of my follow-up sessions.

'Yep', she says thoughtfully, regarding my right side. 'That needs to be fixed'.

And so the third surgery that I was not planning on is planned.

I occasionally wrestle with myself about whether I should just leave things as they are. A third surgery is the last thing I feel like adding to my already overstressed body. And yet, I know that better results are possible. The two women I know who had Bill as their plastic surgeon for post-mastectomy reconstruction both glowed about their results. Words such as 'perfection' and 'masterpiece' were thrown around. Clearly someone has to be the exception that proves the rule, and unfortunately it is me. But I want to feel that at least I have given it the best try possible. So my decision is made. One more surgery and then whatever it is, it is.

30 October 2012

I approach this surgery with leaden feet. On the one hand I feel that unlike the other two, it is the surgery that need not have been necessary. And on the same hand, whereas I went into the previous surgeries trusting that Bill would do an excellent job, now I am not so sure. My spirits are dragging as much as my feet as I yet again walk through the hospital doors.

There is the same ritual of arriving in civilian clothes to the outskirts of the operating theatre – the lively boots, the heated blanket and the meet-and-greet series of pop-in introductions. And then I am wheeled into the operating theatre.

It is the same operating theatre I have been wheeled into twice already this year. Its arrangement is identical to that of my previous visits. As is my position on the trolley. And yet, suddenly, for the first time in all of my operating theatre visits, my glance falls upon an array of sharp, glittering, surgical steel. The instruments. It is impossible to see them and not immediately think of what they are about to do to my body. I avert my eyes. I am utterly startled. They have clearly been there on every visit I have made and yet I have never seen them before. And then I realise that this is the first visit on which I have been wheeled in without having total trust in my surgeon. And that trust has protected me from this sight.

The surgery takes two hours. I wake as usual in my room. But this time with a difference. In order to fill the dents and ridges, small amounts of fat need to be taken from other sites in my body and injected into the dents. The areas from which the fat has been taken need to be compressed. Enter the surgical compression garment.

The surgical compression garment is my nemesis. I hate it with a passion. The constriction makes me nauseous, the hard edges rub against my skin and it is a 24/7 deal for the next four weeks. I think about burns patients who have to wear these kinds of garments for months on end and I feel faint at the thought of how unbearable it must be.

A friend tells me that she tried on some euphemistically named 'shapewear' at the urging of another friend. In the fitting room she managed to tug on this modern-day version of the corset and nearly had a panic attack on experiencing its escape-proof, all-encompassing super-constriction. She turns pale as I describe my surgical garment fitting, where the first question the fitter asks me, after the zips have been finally, impossibly, squeezed closed, is 'Now, can you breathe?'

And then, an hour later, as I flick through a magazine lying around, I come across an article by a woman who had all-over body liposuction. I scream inwardly at the very thought, knowing that all-over liposuction means all-over compression garments. And yes, as I read on, there she is describing them. 'I found them rather cosy and comforting', she says. And as I do a double-take the equivalent of two backward-pike somersaults, I realise that it does indeed take all sorts.

14 November 2012

I am given early release from my prison garments and allowed out of them after two long, long weeks. The relief I feel at being compression-free is tempered with an odd fleeting guilt akin to skipping school and being caught truanting. I have been so focused on having to serve out the four-week sentence Bill has given me that to suddenly have it commuted to two weeks feels unnerving. This is also partly due to the doom-laden words of a nurse who instructed me on all the terrible things that would happen if I didn't wait out those four weeks. Mostly, however, I am just amazed, exhilarated and boundlessly appreciative of being free of the wretched things.

There is something anticlimactic about the third surgery. Or rather about the idea of the third surgery. A 'been there, done that' notion. My body, however, is not buying into that nonchalance. It is letting me know without reservation that it does not appreciate having three major surgeries inflicted on it within the space of eight months. I am far more tired than I expected to be. And the date on which I optimistically opted to go back to work arrives much more rapidly than anticipated.

Over the next few weeks, I have the strangest sense once again of leading two split, parallel lives, one as the patient who is just catching her breath and one as my competent self. Slowly, very slowly, as the year moves on, they begin to merge into one.

2 February 2013

The surgeries seem a long way behind me – a distant part of my life. My body is my own again, although it is a different body. I don't think of my breasts, they are simply there.

With a mastectomy, nerves have to be cut, meaning there is no sensation left in the reconstructed breasts or unreconstructed chest area. I have expected this – it is part of the price paid for safety. Before my surgery, a woman on the FORCE website had posted her concern that with no nerve endings in her breasts, she would be unable to feel hugs from her daughter. This was one of the 'side effects you don't expect' that had stuck in my mind as I tried to imagine a world in which you could not feel hugs. To my relief, however, hugs feel the same and are just as wonderful as they were before surgery.

The other unexpected side effect I had read about – pectoral muscles that shiver in the cold, resulting in visibly vibrating breasts, has also not eventuated. As I am regularly called upon to give lectures in the winter, I am deeply grateful that this side effect has not come about either.

25 March 2013

It is more than three-and-a-half years since Martin's stroke and five months since my last surgery. I am myself again, back doing and being all the things I think of as 'me'. I have still had no chance for a holiday – a manuscript deadline and an extra-large caseload of patients do not mesh with a relaxing, no-responsibilities spot of R and R, but I am feeling as if the world has normalised.

It is, in fact, feeling so normal that it is hard to recall the terror of that time, the ripping away that made me want to go running out into the street, waving my hands and shouting, 'Don't you understand? Open your eyes. You have to see. Everybody dies. That's what it's about. The people we love die!'

I have also started writing poetry again. And remembering how much I love it. Whereas when I write prose of various kinds I feel as if I am talking, thinking or meditating out loud, when I write poetry I feel as if I am dreaming out loud. The poems are about Martin's illness. Throughout these three years, words have been emerging from me in strata – first through emails, then the prose of memoir and then poetry. It feels luxurious to be digging in the rich, deep earth of poetry again.

Martin is wonderfully well – doing all the things he loves, speaking with his new accent and displaying more energy and stamina than I possess. My surgery scars are healing nicely. The surgeries seem far away. I don't think about them now unless I come across a particular mention of the BRCA gene or mastectomy. The future seems to stretch out again – it seems foreseeable and stable. Martin and I are in it, as are Amantha, the people we love and Harriet.

I have finished work and am getting ready for bed when the phone rings. It is a friend and he is phoning to tell me that a treasured friend we have all known for decades has just suddenly and unexpectedly died. I can tell he is having difficulty believing the words as he speaks them, just as I am having difficulty understanding them.

This friend was fit and healthy – playing enthusiastic tennis a few days ago with no hint of sickness. We have all seen him recently and he was his usual energetic self. It is impossible to think of him dead. The concept keeps sliding off my mind. It is oil to water – there is no way it can be absorbed.

A few of us in this group of friends have had illnesses. This friend did not. It seems insane to think that one day you can be vital and full of life and the next day dead. And I realise that in my mind there has been an addendum to the belief that we are all going to live forever. It is that 'and if we don't live forever, we will get sick first'. There will be treatment and chances, remissions and recurrences. There will be surgery and drugs that add time. And there *will* be time. Time to get used to ill health. Time to talk. Time to gather resources. Time to prepare. Time to understand. Time to be there. Just time.

In the morning, in between patients, I go for a walk. It is sunny – Melbourne has thrown up blue skies and an excess of light. My friend's face keeps appearing in front of me. His mischievous smile, his quick intelligence, his quirky wit and the soft voice that you had to listen to closely. How can he have just vanished? And I alternate between believing that he has and believing that he has not.

And once again, I am plunged into that split sense of reality. Part of me is walking in the sunshine, healthy and normal and familiar. And the other half of me is walking in that other world. The door clicks open and clicks closed. I am here and I am there. And sometimes I am in the doorway.

Years ago, during an idle conversation with a friend about favourite words, I volunteered that one of my favourites was 'interstitial'. She looked at me with eyebrows raised. Trained in the biological sciences, she was used to thinking of 'interstitial' as referring to a space in a tissue or body part, such as the space between the veins of a leaf or an insect's wing. For me, interstitial was simply 'the space between'. I loved it, along with its companionate word 'liminal', the word taken from *limen*, the Latin for 'threshold', which means being at or on both sides of a boundary or threshold. Both 'interstitial' and 'liminal' sing of freedom – the freedom to define yourself, to explore, to be one thing or the other, the freedom to shift between worlds, perspectives, to cross boundaries, to create and to recreate. What could be wrong with words like these?

I had forgotten that 'interstitial' and 'liminal' are also the defining words of the Trickster gods. The Trickster appears in the mythology of every culture. His names are myriad: Hermes, Loki, Enki, Maui, Eshu, Anansi, Coyote and that wonderful bird the Raven.

The Trickster lies and cheats. He is amoral, has huge appetites and doesn't care how he fulfils them. The Trickster misbehaves, breaks rules and conventions, even the most sacred. He is unfair. He often makes a fool of himself, and always makes a fool of others. The Trickster loves mess and chaos. He leaves a trail of collateral damage he barely notices and if he did he might not care. He is what we do not want our children to be and yet the Trickster tales are the ones told to children all over the world. Adults love the Trickster stories too. Even in the twenty-first century in the Western world, we celebrate a festival dedicated to the Trickster – April Fools' Day or All Fools' Day, when we play pranks on unsuspecting people to fool them, disrupt them, take them by surprise.

The Trickster is the definition of paradox. He destroys thoughtlessly but he also brings gifts. He gave us the sun and the moon, fire and fishing nets, even as he brought us Death. He is the storyteller who gave us language, which can be used either to tell the truth or to deceive. He is one of the few allowed to move between the heavenly realms and the Underworld, from which no one else returns. He is the lord of misrule but just as surely the lord of creation. He lives in doorways, boundaries, crossroads, on the edge. He lives between here and there, between right and wrong, between this and that. He changes, he shapeshifts, his natural habitat is uncertainty. He lives in even the smallest spaces between atoms. Heisenberg's uncertainty principle is the principle of the Trickster. He cannot be pinned down.

He is infuriating, childish, a troublemaker – everything that drives us wild – but he is necessary. Trickster is a low-life, a tramp and a tinker, but he is also the engine driving the world. Trickster frequents the rubbish dumps everyone else avoids. The ones we all have. The ones that contain everything we have discarded, that we are sure we do not need, that we are disgusted by, that we are frightened of – everything we have banned, burned, thrown out, dumped somewhere beyond the limits of our well-groomed cities.

Trickster has no home – he is of the road – a traveller, a mover, an itinerant – but the trash heap is where he comes again and again. This is where he is most surely at home – among the objects that have lost their assigned function, the pairings that are haphazard, the mess that is wonderfully, brilliantly random. Trickster will find something in there. He is the god of the unexpected, the transitional and ultimately the transformational. Trickster loves mess and chaos. Trickster would linger in op shops. Their very name, after all, stands for opportunity – something for which Trickster has a genius. All those discarded, less-loved, given-away objects waiting for Trickster to flip, strip, bring into their new life. Trickster kicks us out of stasis. He makes life happen.

There are innumerable Tricksters in popular story and myth – Puss in Boots, Brer Rabbit, Reynard the Fox, Prometheus and, perhaps the wiliest of all the Trickster heroes, Odysseus, whose legend is as vibrant today as it was thousands of years ago. I loved them all as a child. I fell in love with the Greek myths in Arthur Mee's *Children's Encyclopaedia*, discovered the Norse myths, devoured fairy tales and folktales from every source I could find. I read under the covers when I was supposed to be asleep, I read in the bumpy backs of cars where my father drove as though he were king of the road, and I read in a different motion while walking to school. I read everything I could read. But there is always one story where the reader's eye drags.

For me it was the Grimm brothers' tale 'The Story of the Youth Who Went Forth to Find What Fear Was'. It is the story of a young man who 'could neither learn nor understand anything'. He notices that while others scare themselves by the fire at night – shuddering at the tales of ghosts and monsters – he does not shudder. When the time comes for him to start earning his keep, all he wants to do is learn how to shudder.

Throwing his hands up at his son, but imagining that it will be easy to teach him to shudder, the father arranges for the sexton to dress as a ghost and frighten him. The youth is not frightened, however – all he sees is a man dressed in a white sheet.

He sets out on the road, still seeking fear. A passer-by tells him to spend the night by the gallows on which hang seven corpses. But the youth does not realise they are dead – he only wonders that they are so cold and is irritated that they will not warm.

Successive attempts to frighten him all meet with the same results – nothing can give him the shudders. Finally, he meets the king who has promised his daughter in marriage to the man who can spend three nights in a haunted castle. The castle is inhabited by ghosts and demons, and many men have entered but none have returned.

The youth spends three nights there and is accosted by the castle's ghouls and spirits but fails to recognise how terrifying they are, deals with them matter-of-factly and emerges unscathed. The astonished king is forced to give him his daughter's hand in marriage.

He is settled now, wealthy and married to a princess. But no matter how happy he is, the youth continues to bemoan his inability to feel fear, constantly crying, 'If I could but shudder. If I could but shudder'. Finally, his new wife takes pity on him, creeps up on him while he sleeps at night and empties a bucket of water filled with cold, slippery fish all over him. As he wakes shuddering, he exclaims 'Ah, now I know what it is to shudder'.

The cheat of this ending infuriated me even as a child. How could the shivers of repellent cold be equated with the shivers of terror? To have spent the whole story searching for fear only to be satisfied with a few cold fish – how could that possibly make sense? And I discarded the story, only remembering it on odd occasions because it had such an interesting title. And there it remained – in the rubbish tip – until now, just now, when the Trickster tossed it up to me.

'Here', he said. 'This is what you wanted. Take this. This is a life without fear'.

And it is. It is the anti-Trickster story. It is the story of not being wholly human – of being without imagination. Of being without the notion of loss. Without the notion of future pain. Without the notion of heartache. And equally surely, without the notion of love. Because once we have loved, we must also understand the fear of that love being taken away.

And love, it seems, is also what the Trickster rules. We do not walk staidly and steadily up to love – we fall into it, trip over it, wander blindly into it. Love makes everything look different even though nothing has changed. Love makes us better people. Love makes us do terrible things. Love makes us strong. And love is our weakest link. We sing anthems to freedom and with the same voice happily declare our heart hostage. Love is a state of insanity – the neuroscientists have confirmed it. And love is what makes us most sane, the most ourselves and the most a part of something larger than ourselves.

And I am tossed back to the Trickster. This time it is Loki, the Norse god, the archetypal Trickster. I remember his name from childhood because his was another of the stories that filled me with indignation.

In Asgard, where the Norse Gods live, the most loved god of all is the shining one – Baldur the Beautiful, the summer god, son of Odin and Frigg. Baldur is as wise as he is beautiful and as eloquent as he is good. He is the god of truth and light and no lie can pass through the walls of his palace of Breidablik. One night, however, Baldur has the first of a series of terrible dreams – dreams of his own death. Only the truth can exist within the walls of his home. His dreams must be taken seriously.

Frigg, his mother, is determined to protect her son. All around the nine worlds she goes, asking every little and last thing to swear it will never hurt Baldur. All do so. All but the one she has neglected – the mistletoe plant. It is too young, too unimportant, too unthreatening to bother with. Loki the Trickster, however, can be bothered with it.

The gods have a game they play. Knowing that Baldur cannot be harmed by any object, they hurl things at him – for the sheer sport of seeing the rock, the spear, the shard bounce harmlessly off him. Loki, however, has fashioned a spear from the mistletoe that has made no promise to protect Baldur and he has given it to Baldur's blind brother to throw. Unaware of what he has been handed, he throws and Baldur is killed.

How could this be? Reading it as a child, I am beside myself with agitation. How could the god who was only good be killed by the jealous troublemaker? How could they let this happen?

And there it stays. Until I come back to it as an adult years later, many years later – today in fact – and read the story again.

And what I am drawn to this time is not Baldur's glittering goodness. Not Loki's subversive mischief. What I am drawn to this time is the character of Frigg. The mother who sees that terrible things are going to happen to the son she loves. The mother who is desperate to protect him. Who journeys around all of the nine

299

worlds, exacting promises. The mother who is determined to defeat entropy and decay and all of the forces, weak and strong, close and distant. The mother who is going to stop time, as we all want to stop time, suspend it, freeze it to a snapshot, keep it static, handcuffed to when everything is good and the ones we love are whole and happy. Frigg is the mother who has to fail.

And at last I see it – this is why Loki did what he did. Whatever he thought, whatever the impulse, this was Loki's job. Loki is the Trickster. And the Trickster is here to keep the world going. Stasis is not allowed. Stasis is death. Stasis will kill everything. The world has to keep moving.

And it does. It will. With or without us. Loki will be caught and punished. The gods will die in the terrible final battle of Ragnarok. The great old gods will die, but there will be survivors. Two humans who will repopulate the earth. A few gods who have lived through the fighting and those, including Baldur, who will be reborn after it. All will come to this impossible new world rising from the seas, its fields and woods green, its forests filled with wildlife, its skies with birds. And they will live there. They will live.

But before all this, there is Baldur's funeral. As he finally farewells his son, Odin the king of the gods, bends and whispers one word in his ear. What word? What did he say? It is a riddle. No one knows. By the Viking age it has become a common expression for the unknowable. But the old, now long-lost children's book where I first read this story knows. I can see it now. On the page facing the black-and-white illustration, at the end of the rows of paragraphs printed in the old-fashioned typeface on the creamily thick pages, is the sentence at the very end of the story. I can see it clearly. And at the end of that sentence, the end of the very last sentence, is the very last word. The word that Odin whispered. And the word is 'rebirth'.

After the Hospital Room

1 Stone Soup.

*'Stone Soup' is an old folktale in which a hungry traveller tricks villagers
into adding their vegetables and seasonings to a pot that contains only water
and stones. He makes them believe that the resulting soup is a great delicacy
that owes its delicious flavour to the stones in it.*

Before the story
there is always no
beginning. It makes itself
up out of no thing,
the way magicians do,
the way you make stone
soup: Start with a traveller –
soldier, sailor, tinker or simply
someone who has not agreed
to stand still.
He has a cooking pot the way
the sea has basins
and a need to fill.
Begin with nothing. Add
what they give you.

2 The Hospital Room.

You are going where the mountains go
when they pull the clouds closed
for privacy and move the great roots
of their legs like old, old ladies,
forgotten and enormously powerful.
They have their firs as collars and the birds
click around their wrists
like watches. Crazy
as any saint, they remember
all of the names for healing,

and all of the words mean change.
In your hospital room
the sky stayed absolutely normal.

3 **Why the Sky Left.**
Too much harmony can kill
they tell you
in African stories –
Mother was the Earth
and Father the Sky,
all blue with logic,
and so nice to each other
they were barely apart –
would never separate.
They were too good,
the way truth never is
and in love
with safety –
and you know what they say
familiarity breeds.

When the old woman,
call her Mischief,
call her Maker of Things,
call her The One Who Stirs
Us Up, discovered
that she liked the taste of blue -
sky, inky, azure, china, duck-egg,
Prussian too - she reached up and plucked it.
Wouldn't you? Real as a piece of the moon,
soup for two.

Finally angry, the Sky flew
up over our hairdos, blew through
ravens, egrets, Arctic terns,

passed even the bar-headed geese
and further still,
so far above us
that no one could touch it,
stayed like a shrew.
Mother cried, but the rivers
were old news – we had to learn
to make do.

4 Names.
Once I said I loved the word
'liminal', thinking interstitial,
in between, a space, a crack, a place
between boundaries, unrestricted,
no definition, the place that Schrödinger's cat
lives in. I wasn't thinking.
I was forgetting that
these are the words ruled by you
Hermes, god of the Tricksters,
and your colleagues
Loki, Iktomi, Coyote, Crow,
Raven, Anansi, Azeban –
all of them
being of the crossroads
where what you never
know will happen
and interstitial
is a hospital room
where the chip
of Loki's arrow breaks free
and flies to your brain.

5 Labyrinth.
Place of the first dancing.
The bull, the blood, the double-axed
Goddess all live here. Mother of the Earth,
Mother of the blind and terrible
butterfly that tears itself
apart to renew. Mother of the dark.
Mother of the strange
white coming into daylight.
Mother of the upraised arms.
Mother of the new.
Mother of the old
silence.

A labyrinth has only one way
in and the same way out,
which is different. They say the brain
is a labyrinth, telling itself
stories – choices
you think you have found.
Once inside, you must move slowly,
there is an art to this.
Whatever you believe,
they have let you enter
the sound of yourself
walking. The chords of your heart
are growing backwards.
Do not follow.
Unleaf to the centre.
Only then
will they let you leave.

6 Story.

Light is the stars' story
speaking backwards.
It has passed by Altair,
Aldebaran, Askella, Errai.
It has come in a single line
like a good schoolgirl
carrying its files,
its lists of names,
the old, old stories.
What does it do
when your eye stops
it at the soft deceptive border
between what is you and what
is not? Do you become
the story
teller or the told?

7 Odysseus.

Descendant of rustlers.
No wonder Hermes liked you –
cattle-stealing was a family game.
Odysseus, Ulysses, liar, lawyer, talker, story
man. Owner of the name your father
gave you – *Giver and receiver*
of pain.

What did you learn
out there in the stuck eternal
airport of the dead?
The silent
hordes – the lost, gaunt people
of abandoned luggage, surging
forwards, begging,
begging you for voices.

There is not enough blood.
And the story doesn't pause
even though you pray it does.
There is a price for names
And no one's costs more than the one
you give away.

Now, twenty years since the Trojans
woke from nightmare to the morning
horse. The sea blinking and emptied,
the beaches free and nothing
but a single pleading Greek
telling them what they wanted
to believe. And you're on
your final ship.
Everything stowed,
you, the eternal vigilant,
are asleep when they carry you
back to Ithaca
down to the once-familiar
beach. You wake alarmed, befuddled,
sure this is the wrong entry,
scream at the misted shore and run
into the age-old problem
of understanding
how to know
where home is.

8 Stone Soup.
When you write a poem,
you have absolutely no idea
of where you are going
or how it will take you.
Start with nothing.
Make what you find.

APPENDIX

Knowledge about the brain has been changing at an astonishing rate. Fifteen years ago doctors and psychologists were routinely taught that while a child's brain was still plastic – that is, capable of changing and growing – by adulthood the brain was fixed and immutable, incapable of growing new neurons, repairing damage or finding ways to circumvent the effects of damage. We were taught that stroke patients would have a period of recovery that would cover the months after a stroke but that by the time a year had passed no further recovery was possible. This is what doctors and psychologists had been taught for decades. It was knowledge set in stone.

The research on brain plasticity, which has only filtered through to the mainstream in the last decade or so, was not only ground-breaking, it was the equivalent of a major earthquake, upsetting everything that had been known and taught so confidently about the brain's ability to recover from damage. It opened the floodgates to a whole new field of study and research has been pouring through.

Much of this research – good, peer-reviewed research that has not yet filtered down into daily practice – is out there in the form of papers and articles that can be accessed through the internet and libraries. It is so new that it is not yet taught in medical or psychology courses. It is presented at conferences or published in journals, but if therapists are not at the conference or have not read the journals, they may not have heard about it. The reality these days is that with so much information out there it is impossible to read every journal article or go to every relevant conference. Clinicians rely on information being passed down through the system and this takes time. You may not have the luxury of that time.

I was fortunate in that I had the training to understand that research, evaluate its usefulness and think about how to put it into practice. Many would not be able to do so but in that case, there may be people to turn to. Postgraduate neuropsychology students might be happy to earn some money canvassing the latest research on neuroplasticity and printing it out for you. The therapists at your hospital – speech therapists, physiotherapists, psychologists, doctors – might be happy to look at the relevant papers and decide if there is anything they can implement for your benefit. If you have friends who are scientifically trained in the health sciences, they too may be willing to look over the research for you.

I subscribe to a free online service, Science (Health) Daily, which sends a daily summary of selected new research from peer-reviewed medical journals to my computer. Many useful articles on the latest stroke research make their appearance in this goldmine of a digest. It also has searchable archives in which you can locate articles on a particular topic. I also subscribe to *Scientific American Mind*, another treasure trove of cutting-edge information. There are also several books out now on the subject of neuroplasticity. *The Brain That Changes Itself* by Dr Norman Doidge, an instant bestseller, provides an inspiring tour of the field and the exciting developments in our knowledge of brain plasticity.

In evaluating any research, several issues are of paramount importance. First, check that it is published in a peer-reviewed medical journal. This gives confidence that the study design is acceptable and the results have some validity. Secondly, look at whether any harm could come from applying the study's findings. If medication is involved, clearly this has to be discussed with the patient's doctors. Other interventions, such as listening to music, would seem to have no negative side effects if the patient is happy to go along with them. Thirdly, always check with your patient's medical team when adding any intervention. Unless they think it involves dangers or unpleasant side effects, they will usually be happy to go along with it.

A sense of optimism was also a crucial part of Martin's journey. Recovery from stroke involves an immense amount of steady, repetitive work. Results are seen via cumulative small successes that sometimes seem minuscule – optimism and the belief that your work is indeed leading to achievable goals helps you go on. My ongoing reassurance – stressing that Martin's brain could adapt and change – and the encouraging messages on his hypnosis tape were all part of Martin's belief in his goals. He was simply frustrated by his slowness in achieving them.

Depression is a very common companion in the post-stroke period – one study estimated that thirty-three per cent of stroke patients suffer from depression during their post-stroke recovery. Depression is particularly common with strokes that damage the left hemisphere of the brain (the hemisphere usually concerned with language). It is crucial to spot depression in stroke patients and treat it. In addition to the need to circumvent depression, one of the exciting new developments in neuroscience is the discovery that some antidepressants are also in fact associated with neurogenesis – that is they spur on the growth of new brain cells – exactly what is needed in a brain that is trying to repair itself.

It also helps to be assertive within the hospital system. A few years ago, the Dana-Farber Cancer Institute in the United States established a campaign aimed at empowering patients and relatives. They put up posters featuring the slogan 'Check, Ask, Notify' on posters to remind people to participate. Patients and relatives were encouraged to do such things as ask what medication was being administered, check the reasons and the dosage, ask staff to wash their hands before touching the patient if they had neglected to do so, and so on.

More than 2,000 patients were asked about their experience following this campaign. The survey asked patients about their illness, how often they spoke with doctors and nurses about it, whether they had relatives or a friend to help them make decisions and express their wishes, and if they ever checked things such as the medication they were being given. When the researchers looked at their medical records, they found that patients who scored highly on these measures had half the rate of 'adverse events' (mistakes in medication dosage, infection, and so on caused by carelessness) in hospital compared to those patients who hadn't been encouraged to observe and check that correct drug and cleanliness protocols were being followed.

Having been plunged into the role of carer for a very ill, hospitalised patient, I was horrified on a daily basis by the need for my role as patient advocate. Apart from researching the cutting-edge developments in the field, I had the daily tasks of helping to make Martin's life in hospital more comfortable, communicating with the different specialists and therapists to make sure they had the correct current information on

Martin's state, making decisions when different opinions were offered, deciding on the need for second or third opinions – the list goes on. It is horrifying to imagine being as helpless as one is in the wake of a stroke or other serious illness and not have anyone to do that research, advocacy and coaching on your behalf. It is a crucial part of recovery and both Martin and I are certain he would not have had the recovery that he had without my input.

FURTHER READING AND RESOURCES

Brett, Doris, *Eating the Underworld*, Random House, Sydney, 2001
Doidge, Norman, *The Brain that Changes Itself*, Penguin, New York, 2008
Science Daily Health – www.sciencedaily.com
Taylor, Jill Bolte, *My Stroke of Insight: A Brain Scientist's Personal Journey*, Viking, New York, 2007

National Stroke Foundation – strokefoundation.com.au
This national organisation is the only one in Australia that works right across the stroke community. Its extensive network includes healthcare professionals, the research community, stroke survivors and carers, companies and businesses, government and the general public. It has offices in Melbourne, Brisbane, Canberra, Sydney, Perth and Hobart.
National Office: Level 7, 461 Bourke Street, Melbourne, Vic. 3000
Phone: (03) 9670 1000
Fax: (03) 9670 9300
StrokeLine: 1800 STROKE (1800 787 653)

Stroke symptoms
- Sudden numbness or weakness of the face, arm, or leg (especially on one side of the body).
- Sudden confusion, trouble speaking, or difficulty understanding speech.
- Sudden trouble seeing in one or both eyes.
- Sudden trouble walking, dizziness, or loss of balance or coordination.
- Sudden severe headache with no known cause.

Heart Foundation – heartfoundation.com.au
Contact the Health Information Service during business hours for free medical information and support.
Health Information Service: 1300 36 27 87 (cost of a local call)

Heart and Stroke Foundation of Canada
www.heartandstroke.com

American Stroke Association
www.strokeassociation.org

Stroke Association United Kingdom
www.stroke.org.uk/

FORCE: Facing Our Risk of Cancer Empowered
www.facingourrisk.org
FORCE was founded on the principle that no one should have to face hereditary breast and ovarian cancer alone. It is the only national non-profit organisation dedicated to improving the lives of individuals and families affected by hereditary breast and ovarian cancer.
Office: 16057 Tampa Palms Blvd W, PMB #373, Tampa, Florida 33647
Email: info@facingourrisk.org

The Australian Society of Hypnosis (ASH)
www.hypnosisaustralia.org.au
Membership of this society is restricted to qualified health professionals such as psychologists and doctors. ASH directly provides training in hypnosis for any professional who holds registration with the Australian Health Practitioner Regulation Agency. The society views hypnosis not as an independent science but as an adjunct to the range of treatment modalities for a wide range of medical, psychological and dental applications.
National office: PO Box 3009, Willoughby North, NSW 2068
Phone: (02) 9747 4691
Fax: (02) 9747 4375
Email: ashltd@optusnet.com.au

Mirror boxes

These may be purchased from the NOI Group (Neuro Orthopaedic Institute) – www.noigroup.com.

Office: 19 North Street, Adelaide City West, SA 5000

Phone: (08) 8211 6388

Fax: (08) 8211 8909

Email: info@noigroup.com

ACKNOWLEDGEMENTS

One of Stephen Sondheim's songs takes its hat off to the very special grace of old friends. And Lynne B, Elaine, Celia, Denise, Davida and Evelyn, are among the best you could have. As are Cindy and Margot, who, when the three of us first met, managed to spend a year in Luxembourg without ever setting set foot in the country. And of course, there are the twelve special friends of the play-reading group, who have been together so long that we've read some plays three times. And what's worse, not remembered them. And thank you to Ros and Judi, whose 'care parcels' of food were truly gifts of caring from their big, generous hearts. Vivienne B., Ruth, Miron, Carol, Richard, Lynne W., Walter, Eva and Shannon were all there with caring and support in their own special ways. As were our warm and supportive friends from the dance community. And a thank you to Debbie Golvan my literary agent and Terri-ann White my publisher for their belief in, and enthusiasm for, the manuscript in its early stages.

And finally an appreciative acknowledgement of the doctors, nurses and allied health professionals whose expert care was such an important part of the journey.

The real names of hospitals and doctors have been changed throughout this book.

The Neighbouring Bed in the Neurology Ward was shortlisted for the 2012 Newcastle Poetry Prize and published in its 2012 anthology *Coastline*.

CPSIA information can be obtained at www.ICGtesting.com
Printed in the USA
LVOW11s1612241114

415327LV00003B/724/P